BODYBUILDING

Nutrition to Stimulate Maximal Muscle Growth

(The Complete Blueprint to Building Muscle With Weight Lifting)

Lavon Lirette

Published By Simon Dough

Lavon Lirette

All Rights Reserved

Bodybuilding: Nutrition to Stimulate Maximal Muscle Growth (The Complete Blueprint to Building Muscle With Weight Lifting)

ISBN 978-1-77485-310-8

ISBN 978-1-77485-310-8

Legal & Disclaimer

The information contained in this book is not designed to replace or take the place of any form of medicine or professional medical advice. The information in this book has been provided for educational and entertainment purposes only.

The information contained in this book has been compiled from sources deemed reliable, and it is accurate to the best of the Author's knowledge; however, the Author cannot guarantee its accuracy and validity and cannot be held liable for any errors or omissions. Changes are periodically made to this book. You must consult your doctor or get professional medical advice before using any of the suggested remedies, techniques, or information in this book.

TABLE OF CONTENTS

Introduction

In our hectic world it can be difficult to maintain the routines we need to follow to maintain our health. We're always rushing between jobs that we be unable to find moment to workout. However, that's not all of it. It's possible that we're not motivated or may find that exercise is too overwhelming in the sense that we don't know what to do, the reason we should take it up, or what to do first. How do we come up with a solution that is suitable for us? What are the advantages and disadvantages of various methods and equipment?

The next chapters will cover exercises for strength, the most effective method to build muscle without adding fat as well as the scientific basis behind building muscle as well as other useful items. This is where you will learn about the kind of food choices can assist you in reaching what you want to achieve (bet you didn't even know that foods could aid in your workout routine did you? Well, it's true!) The importance of stretching prior to workouts, the distinction between low and high intensity cardio exercises, and many more. This article is intended to inspire and educate you. It's our goal that you be able to use it.

There are many books on the subject available that are available; thank you to everyone who chose this book! We have made every effort to ensure that the book is packed with as much valuable information as we could, so please take advantage of it!

Chapter 1: Beginning The Journey

You've made the decision to take a dip in the waters of bodybuilding.

You're awesome!

You've managed to navigate away from the stereotypes as well as the myths and eye-rolls that could have been greeted by your new love affair. You're about to learn something completely amazing and significant. . .

Bodybuilding is a sport that is a rewarding experience that will provide you with an array of benefits that go beyond the feeling of achievement that comes with winning a contest.

There are also amazing health benefits for your internal body, the part that people don't even be able to. The cardiovascular system of your body will be working well, your joints, bones as well as your immune system be healthier. In addition you'll begin to appear stunning from the outside. You'll also be stronger. This means you'll be less prone to injuries and more prepared to face the challenges of life. All of this can make you wonder why did not jump into bodybuilding many years ago!

But wait! There's more. Training for bodybuilding can help develop essential mental abilities that can improve all aspects of your life. You'll become more determined, more focused and disciplined, and will be capable of overcoming obstacles in your way to success.

In the end, bodybuilding will help you become a fitter and healthier, more attractive stronger, mentally tougher person. Let's begin in this quest . . .

What Are You Now?

The first step in your bodybuilding journey is to take note of where you're at in the present. It's similar to those tests you had to take in school. It's important to learn what you need to know:

Your raw weight

Your lean body mass

The percentage of fat in your body

The main body measurements you need to know about (chest, waist upper arms, thighs, chest calves)

You'll need to buy the best scales. Ideally , your scales should come with a built-in body-fat function. If not, purchase an array of body-fat calipers, and follow the instructions for using the devices. If you're planning on joining the gym, you could anticipate a full exercise and body test during your first workout. Therefore, no matter how you decide to go about it, you'll have to determine the body fat percentage.

When you know your total weight and percentage of body fat, you can calculate the lean mass of your body. Simply multiply the weight of your entire body by the percentage of body fat. After that, subtract the fat percentage from the weight total to determine the lean mass of your body.

This is an illustration:

Raw weight = 65 kg

Length of the body-fat ratio = 28 percent

Real Body Fat = 18.2 kg

The Lean Body Mass is 48.8 kg

You know precisely where you're beginning from. You're able to keep track of every ounce muscle growth and also the amount of weight you're losing.

The next step is to get a good tape measure that you can take your essential measurements of muscle. Measure around the middle of the muscle. Be as exact as you can, every centimeter is important.

Machines or free weights

Machines are excellent to help beginners learn good posture and helping them understand how it feels lifting correctly. This is because they help ensure good technique. They also help isolate specific muscles, and are the best way to go for people who are recovering from injuries. However the machines aren't as versatile in the same way as free weights. Its frame does not permit a proper exercise posture for every body type. It also doesn't promote physical strength. Additionally, machines cannot offer anything other than an approximate comparison between the person's strength curves and the curves of resistance for machines.

Recommendations for Workouts

Utilize machines for the initial 6 weeks of your instruction to understand how to do the move

In the next step, choose free weights to perform your most fundamental movements, like squats deadlifts and bench presses

Utilize cables and machines as secondary exercises to allow an isolated muscle

Chapter 2: Tips to Keep From The

Loss Of Muscle

The process of building muscle is never easy and that's the reason. Each of the muscle groups have their own distinct characteristics in terms of exercise for strength.

For the upper part of the body Many people concentrate upon building their biceps. But strengthening the deltoids are in fact what provides the greatest weight to your upper body. Build the deltoids by using barbells. There are exercises that are aimed at strengthening all the muscles in these areas, and hopefully an athlete would build the routine to work on each of them. Here are a few examples:

Chest Exercises

Barbells, flat or Dumbell Bench Press

Decline Barbell

Flat Chest Press Machine

Push-ups

Pec Dec Machine

Incline Chest Press Machine

The dips in parallel bars
Cable Crossovers
Back Exercises
T-bar Rows
Chin-ups
Pull-ups
Lat Pull-Downs
Seated Cable Rows
Machine shrugs
Barbells as well as Dumbell Rows (bent over)
Chest Supported Machine Rows
Shoulder Exercises
Dumbbell, Machine or Cable Machine Upright Raises
Arnold Press
Dumbell, Barbell, or Cable Machine Upright Rows
Overhead Machine Press
Standing Overhead Barbell or Dumbbell Press
Aft Overhead Barbell or Dumbbell Press
Quadriceps Exercises
Dumbell Step-Ups or Barbell Dumbell Step-Ups
Barbell or Dumbell Lunges

The Barbell, or Dumbell Split Squats
Barbell Squats or Dumbell Squats
The Barbell, or the Dumbell Front Squats
Leg Extensions
Leg Press
Machine Squat/Hack Squat
Hamstring Exercises
Leg curls
Hyperextensions
Cable Pull-Throughs
Glute-Ham Raises
Dumbell Romanian Deadlifts or Barbell
Dumbell Romanian Deadlifts
Straight Leg Barbell or Dumbell Deadlifts
Biceps Exercises
Biceps Curl Machine
Cable Curls
Hammer Curls
Concentration Curls
Incline Dumbbell Curls
Standing Barbell and Dumbell Curls
Barbell or Dumbell Curls for Preachers
Triceps Exercises
Bench Dips
Overhead Barbell or Dumbell Triceps
Extensions

Cable Press-Downs
Skull Crushers
Close grip push ups
Decline Close Grip Bench Press
Flat Close Grip Bench Press
Dips

This is not a comprehensive overview of all options at your disposal. To list every machine as well as exercises and routines that the search will result in a list that is unnecessary repetitive. Differentiation could be due to the type of grip, the custom-made adjustments and so on. Other factors. Take note that specific muscles will be focused on in a second way when performing the exercises mentioned above.

Before we can get into the specifics of how to put your routine together it is important to determine the level of your expertise. This is crucial because there are a variety of differences between the various levels of skill according to the skills you're competent at and what you can do to likely be effective for you.

Beginners should stick to their first workout in order to achieve the most effective results.

Intermediates should follow an intermediate training regimen in order for the best results.

Advanced trainees must follow an advanced program.

A beginner is one who has been practicing for less than six months regardless of whether they're doing it in correctly. If you've been practicing it in a way that isn't right for a long period of time, you may have noticed your results were not satisfactory. Perhaps you tried to practice properly, but quit for a period of time. Here are some suggestions to remember: novices should not try to make all sorts of modifications at once which can lead to failure. To form positive habits, newcomers need to make small adjustments in small increments at one at a time. If you're a novice and want to improve your fitness, you'll be able keep going if you begin slowly. Go to the gym at least once a week, and at times. If you aren't feeling like going to the gym nevertheless then go in and return. This will allow you to form the habit of performing your workout routine. One way to know whether you're performing the exercises correctly, is to examine your posture shoulders back and chest out, then stand or sit tall with your abs tight. A good posture is a good form.

When is it appropriate for a beginner to step into intermediate form? If a newbie has been practicing well for 6 months and having impressive outcomes, should they move to intermediate? Not necessarily. A continuation of their first workout could be beneficial to them or more. The length of time should not be the deciding factor rather, use common good sense. Intermediates have gone through an exercise program that helped them develop a baseline level of muscle strength that allows them to work at a higher capacity. They've improved their form until they are near perfect.

Advanced trainees are working at the most advanced fitness level that there is.

In the advanced classes, the athlete is looking for the development of mass and strength by reducing muscle, rebuilding and expansion. Advanced, high-intensity, low rep set are followed by sets that include repetitions that fill the targeted muscles with blood. Training generates waste products in cells, resulting from burning fat and sugar to power muscular contractions. The buildup of waste draws water into muscles cells, stretching the cells' wallsand temporarily increasing the volume of muscle and forming pathways that permit for continuous expansion.

How can you tell at what level you are? Be realistic. If you've never tried exercise, or believe that a treadmill is an unpaved road, you're a beginner. If you've not yet devised an exercise program for yourself or for anyone else, you're a novice. A lot of people rate themselves more than their actual expertise. It's not going to work , not all most of the time but but not all the time. Beginner exercises are designed suitable for novices. The idea of conflating your level of training is to mislead nobody.

It is best to be truthful, and be in the right position so that you know what is the best option for you and help you to move towards your objectives.

In terms of the frequency you need to workout You must decide how often you are likely to exercise every week. This is called your Overall Fitness frequency. The best way to go about it is to do your routine of exercise 3-5 times per week. Take a break throughout the week, but let your muscles to recover. Do not exceed two exercises with weights consecutive days.

The Muscle Body/Group Part The frequency is once every week, twice per week, or 3 times a week. You may have realized that training each muscle group every week is not as efficient than doing them three times or twice each week.

The once-a-week group could include:

Those using steroids/drugs

People who need to keep themselves in the place they are

People who are genetically above average, they can perform once a week what

It takes the majority of people three times a week be successful.

People in the advanced category who are looking to focus on a specific body component

or muscle group

Also, do not include:

Anyone who has a performance or strength goal

People who want to tone up, build muscle or simply look better

In the three times-a-week model the muscle section and body part is exercising once every 2nd or 3rd day which is quite strenuous. Instead of making sure that you are able to provide sufficient training that you are able to take a week off What you need to do is give just the right amount, not excessively and not too small. Too much and you'll not be fully recovered prior to the next session, which is just three or four days later.

It is a common misconception that a change to a three times per week schedule simply involves taking the number of reps and sets that they did at the levels one and two and performing them more often , at least two or three times per week. No. You'll never be able to recover fast enough. Instead, use the same amount and split the weight in a way that is evenly distributed over three sessions.

Who is this three-times-a week scenario suitable for? Anyone who is beginning, regardless of what their purpose is, and everyone who is looking to build strength. This frequency is high enough to allow individuals to develop their motor skills significantly faster.

Do three times a week bring positive results for anyone? Sure however, the issue here is what's most effective for you and what isn't.

Be assured that we haven't completely skipped over the workout twice a week. This routine consists of every muscle group is worked two times a week, on the 3rd or the 4th day. This is an average frequency. Any situation in which each muscle group is exercised at least once every 3rd or 5th day is considered to be a moderate exercise. This has the added benefit of removing the issues that the other two frequencies can bring.

One issue in creating muscles can be whether you should stretch prior to exercising. There are those who believe in it, while others claim that stretching is a cause of injury and this is often the case. But, if done properly stretching should not cause injury or pain. The kind of stretch that we practice and the time we do it, can affect the flexibility. If this isn't happening it is best to check the practice to determine if it is not adequate. When we exercise specific muscle groups get more powerful and shorter. Once the muscle groups have been recognized, a regular program of stretching needs to be designed around them to loosen them up and prepare for a workout. Most commonly, muscles that are tight are located in the front of the thighs (hip flexors) as well as the chest and neck muscles, as well as the hamstrings. If you are stretching, do each stretch for a minimum of 30 seconds with a deep breath. Pause for a second before performing the stretch once more. Repeat the stretch three times. This is a moderate stretching. While you are stretching, the intensity to allow you to stretch out a bit more at a later time.

It is advised to stretch out after working out. The muscles then might be squeezed tight and crunched. When they're stretched, they'll be flexible and open, which means it's a great moment to consume some protein. Protein is a fast-growing protein that spreads quickly throughout these muscles, building strength and bulk.

A lot of people think the stretching as well as warming-up are two different things. However, this is not the case. It is just an attempt to reduce the strength of the stretch, as shown in the illustration above. While it is essential to warm up to avoid injuries, it does not stretch muscles. A gentle warmup in which the participant is jogging or walking for about 10 minutes is enough to increase blood flow to the muscle that is in question. The actual stretch described above should be performed following the warmup or the exercise.

Muscle tissue is distinct. It's composed of three distinct kinds of fibers that are Type I, IIa, and IIb. Different sports produce various fibers. The mix of the three types found in every person's body is different. In general, every athlete is a particular kind, particularly if they are specialized in a specific sports. This is because every type has its own distinct characteristics and is associated with a specific kind of movement. Each type is unique and has the characteristics of a metabolic and contractile and are classified into slow twitch and speed twitch fibers. This does not mean athletes are restricted to only one type of sport, as with diligent training, they can use all three types to be successful in a variety of sporting activities.

Slow twitch fibers appear colored red because of their iron content. They contract gradually, but they can hold their contractions for a prolonged period of time. They are used in endurance events of a long duration that require longer periods of time. This includes race distances, marathons skiers who cross-country, etc. Many, huge mitochondria inside these fibers help in the metabolic process of oxygen. These fibers are able to withstand fatigue, but only produce the force of a small amount.

The count of slow twitch fibres of sedentary children and adults is typically around 50 percent in endurance athletes, while those who train for endurance sports typically contain around 90 percent. The lowest amount of slow twitch fibres, approximately 25%, is present in athletes who rely on brief bursts of energy.

Fast twitch fibres, types IIa and IIb, swiftly transmit energy at a rapid turnover rate, and speedy contracting of muscle. They release calcium quickly. These fibers' properties enable them to release rapid bursts of energy that last for a short time. Sportsmen who play soccer, hockey and basketball, as well as people who exercise and engage with track and field will find these fibers extremely useful. They exert a significant amount of force. are not as resistant to fatigue as well as contract with a greater rate than the slow Twitch kind.

Fast fibers that twitch of IIb type IIb kind are among the least prone to fatigue of the three types, however they also generate large amounts of force. The sports that require an abrupt surge of energy use this type of fiber. However, their effectiveness is short-lived, only lasting 7.5 milliseconds. They are the last ones to be utilized in workout exercises: slow twitch fibers are the first to be used followed by the type IIa after that slow-twitch fiber is running out of energy. Finally, IIb fibers are used to generate maximum power and strength.

A muscle group with muscles with short tendons and long bellies can expand quickly if exercised with the appropriate level of intensity. Muscles that weigh a lot initially will respond quickly to exercise. They also have greater accessibility in the compound exercise. According to the rule of thumb long muscles develop the most rapidly.

For each of these muscles, not all will succeed However, this could be due to the diet or drugs used or other factors. In this case, there might lack the muscle to build.

Chapter 3: Ketogenic Chiseling

The most effective and efficient way to lose weight is to adopt the Ketogenic eating plan. If you're overweight and not utilizing an Ketogenic diet, then you're not going to see outcomes. A Ketogenic eating pattern will cut out every gram of fat that is in your body. It's most effective way to lose weight for those who are obese. A Ketogenic eating pattern is basically zero carbs. Absolutely no carbs or a minimum amount of carbs since the majority of foods contain less than one gram of carbohydrates per portion.

If you follow the Ketogenic eating plan, you won't be eating bread, fruit chips, or anything else that contains sugar, rice, noodles, potatoes pizza, pasta cornbread and corn, as well as nuts that contain carbs and everything else with carbs. The carbs are completely eliminated in your diet. Carbs are the simplest energy source for your body to utilize and when your body utilizes carbs to fuel itself, it doesn't make use of fats and store the fats within your body. If you eliminate carbs from your body, however the fats are utilized as energy sources by your body, and they don't become stored, which results in a loss of fat.

The process of becoming Ketogenic isn't easy , since nearly everything contains carbs today. This is why you shouldn't be doing it long-term. You should stick to the Ketogenic eating plan for a short time and only until you have lost the fat you wish to shed. I'm going to provide you with an Ketogenic eating plan to follow when you're looking to shed weight. This diet plan incorporates intermittent fasting, and you'll only consume two meals a day. Alternate between day 1 and 2 each day until you're happy with the weight loss.

Day 1

The first dinner of the day - Three eggs, cooked with butter. A steak that has been cooked with butter and a few cauliflower.

The second dinner of the day - three eggs in butter cooked, a chicken breasts cooked in butter along with some broccoli.

Day 2

The first meal of the day: Salmon prepared in olive oil cheese, two eggs cooked with butter along with some spinach.

The second meal of the day : Sausages cooked with olive oil cheese, two eggs cooked with butter and a few carrots.

Chapter 4: Bodybuilding Principles

I have never been a fan of following the rules. In fact I have never done so. The good thing is that bodybuilding doesn't have to be about following rules, but rather applying guidelines and principles which provide regular and consistent outcomes. The concepts I will be telling you about are interrelated and you will not be successful by choosing one to adhere to and the other one to disregard. Remember that these aren't methods of training. These concepts may seem stupid, uninformed and evident However, a bodybuilder won't achieve success if they're not observed.

Principle No.1

- Perform every body part at a minimum of every week

It is beneficial to exercise each body part at a minimum of every week. Even those who train every part at least once a week, they should train for it every 5 days. If you're serious about having success quicker, and in the correct way to do it, you have to be ready to put in the effort to attain the desired outcomes. When you combine your willingness with an optimistic attitude to work You will begin to believe that more is certainly better and you'll quickly improve your skills. As a beginner you'll train every portion twice or even three times per week.

The issue is that if the increase in training frequency it can result in a poor recovery. Keep in mind that the purpose is reaping the rewards that recovery brings. Training is a process of stimulating, recuperation and so on.

Once you begin your training, the desire to improve your performance increases, and it is tempting to over-train. The next question is what is the best time to exercise that body part? The real answer is when it is fully recuperated. What time will it take before it is able to recover from the exercise? It's based on various factors , such as the intensity and duration of the training overall.

Here's a basic principle: the more injured the muscle after a workout is, the longer will the recovery.

As you begin your training, it's important to record all your training sessions. They will allow you to see the things that work for you and what isn't. One aspect that could require more tweaking is the frequency of training. Whatever schedule of training you adhere to, it does not mean that it will work for you in 100%. this is the reason you have to find the right appropriate balance between frequency and recovery. This will let you be 100% adaptable.

Furthermore, you must to be aware of the proper expectations. This could mean calves and abs in the back. Abs and calves recover quicker over other parts of the body. This means you shouldn't expect the same results for all body parts. Some parts may require more work than others.

Principle No.2

3-4) exercise for every body component

As I mentioned that it is crucial to strike a balance between the frequency of training as well as intensity of training and the volume of training. This, along with the following one, will aid in controlling the your training volume.

Although there are occasions when you'll perform 1-2 workouts per area, or sometimes even five, it's not an amount of consistent exercise that guarantees the success you want. It is best to be a little more simple and limit yourself to three to four exercises for each body component.

This way you can have a wide variety of exercises to make sure that every muscle is activated in a unique way. This is done by using different exercises, reps and rest intervals. I suggest doing four back exercises, and two each for biceps and the triceps.

Do not imagine the leg is a single muscle group. It's not. It's a collection of muscles, just like calves and hams as well as quads. Do not lie to yourself by doing only 3-4 exercises to strengthen your whole lower body, because ultimately you'll look like an unformed muscular man.

To be a professional bodybuilder is to focus on each muscle individually such as 3-4 exercises for the quads and three for hams and calves. It may at first seem like a lot, especially when you look at the table I'll give to you in the book, but it's not. To become a professional bodybuilder, you must be prepared to be a gruelling training session.

Principle No. 3

3. Practice 3 sets of workouts for each exercise

I've seen and heard numerous people quantify the volume of training and training sessions using total sets. To me, this does not make any sense This is the reason the reason.

Warm-ups should not be included in the training program because they aren't able to recover Instead, you should count those "work exercises." The term "work set" refers to the time closer to the time that you will not be able to perform another rep. Any set that's less strenuous is merely an exercise set that is preparatory.

Principle No. 4

Power and/or strength move
The goal of bodybuilding is to improve the body, not necessarily to be more powerful or powerful. The pursuit of strength and strength is a fundamental part of your bodybuilding workout.

If you are looking to train for greater energy, it's important to perform more work in a shorter time. In this way, muscles will be able to stimulate or recruit an abundance of muscle fiber all at once.

This will increase your power; However, it's also that is unique for bodybuilders. The increased efficiency will draw additional fibers, which will be stimulated and stressed to the point of adjusting or adjusting. In the sense that your muscles will get bigger and more powerful.

The muscles fibers will increase in 10% during a time, and the benefits you reap will be remarkable. Utilizing 3x5 (3 sets five reps) on the push press barbell during your routine will make exercises with the shoulder dumbbell 3x8 reps much more efficient.

Strength and power are about speed and strength. They are achieved by lifting more weight regardless of the speed. This type of strength training provides the same benefits to power training but incorporates muscle fibers too. The effect is the same and will help make the other exercises much more efficient.

Remember that training for strength can lead to hypertrophy, or the expansion of the muscles by developing new myosin as well as actin filaments. However, the total impact of doing high-intensity and low rep sets may not be very impressive when compared to time under tension (time in tension) that is a result of strength training and producing muscles that look dense.

If you're not interested in the performance of your athletics, doing only one strength or power move for each part of your body will create an attractive appearance.

Principle No. 5

For each body part do a hypertrophy/strength workout

When I speak of strength and hypertrophy exercises, I am referring to exercises and sets that have the aim of increasing both strength and hypertrophy. As I mentioned earlier that low-rep sets can increase strength, however with less resistance, and an increased speed, the set with a low rep is the best way to boost power.

The issue is that the low rep sets don't trigger hypertrophy to its maximum. This can be accomplished through extended TUT through the induction of the muscles to undergo metabolic stress.

If you are looking for an exercise that stimulates greater the strength and hypertrophy, it might be best to choose 8-10 reps. This allows you to utilize heavier weights to achieve your hybrid goals, yet lightweight enough to boost the time Under Tension.

Be aware that anything between 6 and 12 reps are fine as long as you don't finish with less than 6 reps since this could affect hypertrophy. If it's about 12 repetitions, this could reduce the strength.

A variety of bodybuilding exercises is essential. If you're looking to pick the most efficient repeat range, you should choose between 8-10.

Principle No. 6

-Do a volumization/endurance exercise

People who enjoy the burning sensation and the maximum pump tend to skip low-rep high sets. Those who prefer lifting heavier do not pay attention to reps in a higher range. Over 12 repetitions are a good way to build endurance, and also provide visual effects due to the more intense sets. Training with higher repetitions will increase the duration of the TUT and thus improve hypotrophy.

When we speak of muscle enlargement and not just muscle fiber, it's known as volumization. The muscle's size increases because of an rise in the number and/or dimensions of mitochondria, capillaries and sarcoplasmic retina enlargement and more.

The best set to increase your volume is an exercise that has 12-20 reps. The result is more rounded and fuller muscles. However, keep in mind that to have bigger muscles, you must to increase the size of all parts of them. If you don't do this, it's similar to putting cash on the counter.

Principle No. 7

Isolation exercises, and use compound

By following this principle it is possible to know which one is best to increase muscle size exercise alone as well as compound exercise. For example, are leg extensions more beneficial or squats preferable for quads?

Each of them has advantages and disadvantages. It is best to exercise your muscles in a variety of ways. This means that you'll see overall hypertrophy through every exercise, rather than doing only isolated exercises or compound.

As a bodybuilder it is important to understand that you shouldn't just perform compound exercises. Sure, it can help you build more strength, but it will not be the result you're trying to achieve in building your muscles.

Isolation exercises may not be really "functional" in terms of practicality, but they will put the emphasis on the muscle you wish to strengthen. It will ensure your muscle is subjected to the correct exercise and tension.

Principle No. 8

Exercise to strengthen your weaknesses

Since bodybuilding isn't only about muscle and training and is also about art, it is crucial to keep symmetry and aesthetics in your mind. Many bodybuilders become entangled in the pursuit of greater performance and then begin doing heavier lifting, performing more repetitions, etc. In some instances, doing both. But, remember that bodybuilding gains won't be achieved by simply increasing your fitness level; rather it's due to improving your appearance.

Consider yourself an artist, and you are creating an aesthetically beautiful body. Here's how you can succeed. Take a photo of yourself, and then look at it the way you would do for others. Cover your head in case it makes it easier to be neutral. Then, you must categorize your body components as weak balanced, dominant, or underdeveloped and then use that to design your training plan and address your weaknesses.

If, for instance, the width of your back is your issue, try exercises that are designed specifically for that area. Keep track of your workouts as it may take time to build your body.

Principle No. 9

Then, perform the essential exercises.

This concept is linked to the one before. What happens when you choose the wrong time for the right exercises? The results could be negated.

If you're trying to improve your back to strengthen it, and you finish the workout last then what happens? Nothing! You'll not have the strength and endurance to increase your weight for more reps in order to work on the weaknesses you have. This means that if have an exercise that is important in your the back of your mind and in your schedule make sure you do it first. When you're exhausted will result in a wasted exercise. It is best to do it before you are tired. the most benefits.

Principle No. 10

Rest and reps are Inversely proportional
The bodybuilding principles come from intuition, which is similar the common sense. However, the reality that reps and rest are in fact inversely proportional not an aspect of it. In fact, it's opposite.

Let's say you've completed three reps during an exercise. When you stop resting and relax, your heart rate and breathing get back to normal. You'll notice that it is not long before the two are back to their normal condition. In fact, you haven't felt any heat in the particular body part after a short TUT. After a minute, you'll be able do another set.

If you do take off after doing 15 reps, you'll require more time (about two minutes) before you can resume and continue until your breathing and heart rate has returned to normal.

It's odd that the perception recovery isn't as accurate. Although these two BPMs are crucial (breaths minutes and beats) but there's something else happening that isn't visible.

When fatigue occurs while doing a high-rep set this is due to the ATP-CP mechanism and an inability to the nerve system. It can take up to three minutes for the parts to replenish and rest before you can perform another set with the same level of intensity.

If you are doing high-tension, low rep set that is designed to boost protein synthesis, it's vital to complete every set with as many repetitions as you can using the weight you are given.

Don't reduce your weight as this will not increase your performance because tension is what creates the strength, which in turn creates larger muscles.

The ability to perform higher reps, even with a longer TUT is not necessary since tension isn't the main stressor, but rather metabolism fatigue. This kind of workout can trigger a different exercise stimulus. Metabolic fatigue will not cause myosin filaments or new actions. Instead, it can lead to the hypertrophy of other structures such as mitochondria, capillaries as well as reticulum and capillaries.

If you are doing heavy, but low-rep sets, make sure you be able to rest for a while to be able to lift the weight you want to during your next workout. The tension causes the muscles to increase in size.

Principle No. 11

Volume and intensity are proportional to each other in an inverse manner

I've set this rule as the number one since it's the most crucial. If you don't adhere to this rule, you will not be able to see any improvement. Many bodybuilders have struggled with this principle the most.

The question is the degree of commitment to giving everything you've got to an exercise. There is a misconception that you should complete as many repetitions as you can. If your life is on it. It is only when you reach that point can you attain the full intensity. In the context of volume, it's the amount of sets, reps, and exercises that you do during a single exercise. This is the number of sets completed until fatigue is reached.

It is crucial to understand that if you're doing all-out sets during one exercise, you need to perform fewer sets overall. If you do not, you'll be weakening your recovery frame.

You can train for long or hard, but you aren't able to train long and hard.

It is best to continue making steady advancement. Train intelligently and not overly. Make use of your new nutrition knowledge as well as the principles that will form your recipe for success in your fitness and bodybuilding.

Chapter 5: Additional Information

Although feeding your body healthy food choices is good however, there are supplements that can help you on your weight-training journey! Beginning with the everyday multivitamin to more sophisticated supplements that are more advanced, we offer you a brief list of the supplements to consider if you want to be female bodybuilders. Keep in mind that these are just suggestions. There is no need for every equipment item we recommend.

Multivitamin

If you're not already taking one, we would recommend an multivitamin. They are packed with the vitamins your body requires which you might not be getting from your diet. These are especially beneficial for women who have a deficit in the vitamins B12, iron and folate departments. Be sure to do your homework prior to heading to the shop as the quantity for multivitamins can vary based on the type of brand.

Fish Oil

Certain studies have shown that individuals benefit from Omega-3 fatty acids in supplements to fish oil. These fats are essential to the development of cognitive abilities and overall well-being. According to research, fish oil could reduce the risk of certain cancers and also help keep chronic inflammation at lower levels. With all the advantages it is suitable for the majority of people and will only benefit your body.

Protein

We mentioned it earlier, if you intend on building up your muscle mass, you'll require protein to help provide energy. If you're tired with eating chicken every day, consider drinking a shake of protein. The shakes are not only useful, they also be delicious tasting and offer more than 25 grams of protein! In addition to this method there are many other recipes you can bake or mix the protein you consume into your daily meals!

Probiotics

If you're not aware that there are good bacteria as well as bad bacteria. For us, the good bacteria are what makes our body is able to process food, and take nutrients. When you consume probiotics, you're aiding your body to acquire the healthy bacteria it needs for proper functioning. Find foods like yogurt and kefir that are rich in Bifidobacterium or Lactobacillus. Probiotics are also available in supplement form however, it is important to make sure it comes of a reliable brand. It is not advisable to introduce anything in your body, as this could be extremely dangerous.

BCAAs

You've probably heard the term thrown around. BCAAs are amino acids of the branched chain. In essence, the three main blocks of proteins are isoleucine and leucine and valine. They are amino acids that aid in protein synthesis and aid in post-workout recovery.

Chapter 6: What to hold A Bar Bell

While performing exercises using the barbell with long handles the bar must be held by hand with about sixteen to 18 inches apart, depending on the length of the pupil's shoulders.

There are two primary methods of holding bar bells. One is called the over grip, where the bell is held with the knuckles on top of the handle bar and the thumb underneath. The other option is that of the under-grip, where the handle bar is resting on the palms of your hands when lifting the bell off the floor. This grip type is shown in Figure 1 and the over grip can be seen in Figure 8.

There are three grips that are suitable for specific exercises. Take a look at Figure 16 and notice it is gripped by turning the palms inwards toward one the other. This is known as the opposing grip that is beneficial when handling heavy bars to help keep it from moving out of fingers. It can be beneficial in the exercises 7, 8 as well as Seven of the Second Course. If you are employing this grip, you must reverse your hands frequently to ensure that you don't get used to doing them all the time using the same hand to the opposite direction (or towards the front like seen in the figure). Another variation is to grip that has both hands on opposite sides of the bar. Take note of the location on the hand of left in figure 8D. This grip can make lifting overhead a little less challenging because it can "cut off" to a great extent by tensing the forearm, and then subconsciously locking the biceps against increasing work that the triceps exert. Additionally to those interested in developing their forearms the same grip can be employed for nearly every exercise covered in this class which will bring more benefits for the inner side of forearms. There is another grip that operates differently and requires less forearm effort when gripping the bar. This is known as the German lock grip or hook grip where you hold the bar with your thumb, then wrap the fingers around the bar. When you are done closing your hand then the third and second fingers will slide over the knuckle as well as the thumb nail, effectively locking your thumb in the bar when you lift it and apply pressure on the bar. This grip is not suggested for exercise, unless it circumstances where the hands are weak and cannot support the weight for long enough to allow the robust back and leg muscles to receive a great exercise. When handling massive weights, the most efficient grip to use is to use this grip with an opposing grip. Look up Figure 16 and imagine you have a right hand that grips the bar beneath the ends of the third and second fingers. The same is true for one's left hand. The user would then not be worried about his grip breaking before his back and leg muscles have reached their limits.

How much weight to use?

There are a variety of factors that influence the weight a beginner must employ. The course is based in accordance with the established theory that multiple repetitions of an exercise can build muscle more than just one or two exercises using a high weight.

To determine the proper starting weight, we're guided by the man's age and height, as well as the weight of his body, his measurements, the position he is in and the amount of times he is able to "chin" at the bar, as well as by his prior experience or lack of experience with fitness training.

We try to always be in our SAFE side. Most of the time, when a student begins Regular Exercise No. 1, he discovers it so easy, the student is enticed to increase the weight. He isn't aware that if he puts on all the weight is possible in the regular Exercise No. 1, he could be exhausted before getting to the end of the regular exercise numbers. 9 and 10, and. Therefore, you should avoid beginning with any weight higher than the weights listed in the Regular Exercise No. 1 unless you discuss it with us.

Another reason to begin for a man who has moderate weight. The exercise should be done correctly. Correct movement and posture is the most crucial part of any exercise. Always learn the right method to complete each exercise. Do not rush to finish a move. Make it slow and do it in the way it was intended to be a muscular effort. When you move quickly, it stops being an effort for physical strength; instead, it turns into an anxious motion. It is never safe for your physical progress. Be aware that a competition for lifting is one thing but lifting weights is another. As a body culturist , your goal is to lift an appropriate amount of weight the maximum amount of times (within an acceptable limit specified for every exercise) you are able to achieve this in the correct manner. The sacrifice of correct posture for the extra weight or the chance to do a few more times delays your results longer and will actually mislead you about your achievements. In this regard I would suggest you draw the figures 7A, 7B, 17, and 30 using an ink that is colored so that you are not at risk of being deceived by these figures.

The correct form requires that you ensure that you decrease the weight to a minimum and lift it to the highest possible level each time you repeat every exercise. This will allow you to develop your muscles fully across their entire range of movement, from extension to contraction and completely eliminate any chance of being slowing or tightening your moves. As in Figure 1 for example maintain the wrist in flexion however, lower the weight until your elbows are straight. When you raise it up as shown in Figure 2 do it with strength of your arms and not through throwing or heaving. In Figure 4 the exercise, Exercise 4 in Figure 21 and Figure 28, do not be satisfied when you have your elbows straight. Lock them in a flash and then give a final shrug using your shoulders to raise the weight to its highest achievable point. Then lower until you reach the beginning position, and repeat.

Make sure to remember when making your weights, remember that a 4' pipe bars weigh five pounds, while the five-foot solid steel bar weighs 15 pounds.

PRELIMINARY EXERCISE n°. 1

To build up the muscles of the abdominal region

Figure A

Set the bell of the bar on the ground and lay flat on your back with feet submerged in middle of bar and hands lifted above the head, in the position shown in Figure A. The hands should be thrown upwards and forward, which will help in lifting the body to position in Figure B. Move as far forward as you can and attempt to get toes to meet without bent knees. This will ensure a full contraction of abdominal muscles.

Repeat this several times. As you get stronger, you should not swing your arms outwards, instead remain in a straight line above your the head while slowly rising to sit up by the strength of your abdominal muscles on their own. This exercise is recommended by people suffering with intestinal and stomach disorders. The growth of the abdominal muscles in the front muscles on the abdominal's front increases the blood flow to the digestive organs, and assists to carry out their usual functions.

Figure B
PRELIMINARY EXERCISE n. 2
The ideal is to stand straight, with your heels
together. Bring the arms up over the shoulders; exhale
as you do so. After that, bend your back and try to
place your toes on the floor with your fingers, but without
The knees are bent to bend. Exhale as you bend
down. Take another inhale to assume that the
In a straight position, arms are stretched over the shoulders.
Repeat the bending motion
and not stopping to rest.
Repeat the process several times. If you fail, repeat the process.
If you experience a feeling of dizziness feel dizzy, you may feel dizzy.

Figure C. This exercise is an excellent conditioning exercise and it is especially beneficial for the abdomen and hips.

PRELIMINARY EXERCISE NUMBER. 3

Exercise with dumb-bells to strengthen your sides

Lean back, and put dumb-bells alongside each other.

Right foot. Then, lean forward, and grab the dumb-bell with your

Your right hand, then straighten it up. Take your feet and stand.

About 8 inches apart, and bend as far as you want to

Can be move to turn to the left (see the figure) and straighten the back

again. After repeating this motion, repeat the

the required number of times to move the dumb-bell

on the left side, and do exercises with the left arm.

Repeat 5 times for the same arm. Using between 25 to

50 pounds.Figure D

PRELIMINARY EXERCISE No. 4 for Abdomen

In a position that is lying on your back supine. As you keep your heels in place and your legs straight, elevate your legs up to a point in a straight line with your body. See Figure E. Lower the legs, repeating the process several times.

Figure E
PRELIMINARY EXERCISE NUMBER. 5
for the Waist Region

Standing straight, one hand on the hips. As illustrated in Figure F in Figure F, bend the knee one at a moment and lift it upwards. Once one foot is replaced on the floor, lift the other. Repeat this several times for each leg.

PRELIMINARY EXERCISE n. 6
For Calf Development

The calf muscle of the leg is among the most difficult part of the body to grow, simply because its structure becomes rigid and brittle due to constant use in walking.

The hardened tissue has to first be broken down before it can respond to growth, which usually requires a lot of work initially. Then, progress becomes satisfying.

The kettle-bell or dumbbell should be loaded at a maximum weight of 40 pounds, and then hold it with one hand. Sit up straight on one leg only. (You are advised to let the fingers of your unengaged hand rest against the rear of the stool or against the wall to help you maintain your balance) Check that the leg you're standing on is perfectly straight. Then, slowly, begin to lift up the toes as high you can. When you are at your maximum height, as shown in Figure G. Keep your position for about a moment, and then lower slowly to the ground, repeating the exercise many times. Perform up to 24 moves before adding 5 pounds, and start with 9 repetitions. Don't forget to exercise both legs.

Figure F
R E G U A L

Figure G

EX E R I S E

There are a few aspects of this exercise that are vital. Many students make the error of trying to bring the bell towards their chest and then pull it upwards in straight lines, putting their elbows to the side as they go about it. This is not a good idea and the elbows must be held by the waist, and the bell must be lifted from the hips up to the chest in a semicircle and with the elbows at in the middle of the circle.

Chapter 7: Do Bodybuilders Need A

High Protein Diet?

To be capable of answering this question, we must first determine what a high-protein diet is. High protein is one which has a higher percentage of protein (by calories) relative with the quantity of carbohydrates or fat that it contains. So, a meal which has 30% carbohydrates as well as 50% protein as well as 20% fat could be considered high protein. In addition the macronutrients profile of this diet is perfect for pre-contest diets.

However, during the off-season it is more crucial that bodybuilders consume a sufficient amount of calories and protein than following an extremely protein-rich diet in general. As we discussed in the chapter entitled, How to Know the Calories in Food is Vital for building on muscle, most people should aim for about thirty calories for every kilogram body mass daily.

With our 80-pound man as an example are aware that the man needs to consume about 2,400 calories a day. Additionally, the majority of experts agree that bodybuilders is required to consume two grams of protein for every kg of weight each day.

So, in the case of an 80-kg man would consume approximately 160 grams of protein daily. This is equivalent to the equivalent of 640 calories (protein is 4 calories per Gram).

As a percentage of his total daily calories (2,400 calories) this is about 26 percent. That means the amount of carbohydrates and/or fat will be greater than the protein content which makes it an average protein diet than a high protein-rich diet!

In response to the question "Do bodybuilders require an energizing diet?' the answer is, yes.

If they are attempting to lose weight in preparation for a contest, they'll consume a diet high in protein however, during the off-season they will not but they'll be getting enough protein.

The most high-protein foods for bodybuilders with a tight budget
Consuming a diet high in protein during the course of your day can be vital for bodybuilders and those who want to get the ideal body. The issue is that high protein foods can be costly, making it challenging for many to afford them.

But, there are healthy, high-protein meals of high quality that are affordable for any budget that means providing your body with all the necessary building blocks needed to develop muscle and function at its best is within ability!

I recently went to the local grocery store located in Perth, Western Australia, and discovered the costs for the highest-quality high-protein food that is cost effective. Because Perth is a costly location to live in, you might be surprised to find that similar items are more affordable for you.

Additionally, we will assess the importance of the high protein food by the fact that it contains 40 grams of "complete" (provides all of the necessary amino acids) protein that is about the amount that many bodybuilders want to consume in all of their meals throughout the day.

Below are the top economical high protein food items.

For bodybuilders who are on a tight budget:

1. Free-range eggs

The free eggs in the range were $4.25 for twelve eggs. Since one whole egg has around 6.5 grams of protein,, you must have six eggs in order to come close to forty grams of protein. That means the price in 40 grams of protein in whole eggs is around $2.12. Of course, if use normal eggs, instead of free-range eggs, it's likely to be less expensive.

Another disadvantage of eating entire eggs is their fat amount. 6 eggs that are whole have about 30g of fat that's too much for one meal.

So, if you take out the yolks (to get rid of the fat) the protein content decreases, and you'll need to eat more eggs which will increase the price.

In Australia there are some stores that sell egg whites in cartons and could be a good alternative. They cost about $7.00 for the 950mls. About 400ml is required to give the 40g of protein that's about $2.94.

2. Tuna

The huge tins of springwater tuna were on sale at the time I visited the store and cost $4.69 for 425 grams. Because 160g of tuna is approximately 40 grams of protein that works out to around $1.76.

Tuna is low in fat and doesn't contain any carbohydrate , unless you purchase the tins of flavored tuna, which can have a higher price.

The biggest issue I have encountered with tuna that is plain can be the flavor. If you're not afraid of eating tuna, you're lucky since it's an extremely healthy, protein-rich source of protein.

3. Cottage Cheese

Low-fat cottage cheese cost $3.29 per 500 grams. With 250 grams providing an average of 40 grams protein,, the price is $1.65.

Cottage cheese is a fantastic supply of the casesin (slow-release protein) and glutamine. This makes it an excellent protein choice for a meal before sleep.

However, as cottage cheese is high in sodium, it's recommended to stay clear of it in the days prior to the event.

4. Whey Protein

Whey protein is considered to be the most prestigious of protein. Prices can vary wildly according to the type of protein, the other ingredients it might contain and the amount that the business spends on marketing!

As a "ball-park" figure, you're likely paying approximately $25 for a kilogram (2.2pouinds) when you purchase the product in large quantities.

Because approximately 50 grams of protein powder containing whey will comprise forty grams of protein it comes to $1.25 which is quite affordable!

There are numerous advantages when using Whey protein. It suffices to that it is a complete lack of carbohydrates or fats, and has significant amounts of amino acids of the branched chain. It's also digested form which makes it an excellent post-exercise or pre-workout protein source.

5. Beans

The beans have been for a long time the top protein source for vegetarians. They're available in tins at $1.06 for 400g. They provide 6.5 grams of protein for 100 grams, you'll have to consume about 1.5 tins to consume the 40 grams of protein you need!

Although it's cost-effective for $1.59 per 40g of protein, and provides an excellent amount of soluble fibre, it'll likely take a long time to consume it. However, it however, it does include a lot of sugars (87 grams!) but it does not supply all your amino acids since it's an insufficient protein source.

6. Mutton

The butcher in the local area near the market sells mutton which is the old meat of sheep. It might be a more difficult to chew, but it's very lean. If you prepare it in stew or a casserole it's fine. If you prefer, you can ask the company to chop it up for you, free of cost.

The best part is that it's actually cheap! It's about $6.00 per kilogram! Because around 200 grams provides forty grams of protein, this is $1.20 per serving. This is the lowest price proteins listed in this article!

Personally, I prefer eating food and not be dependent on shakes, and mutton is a good choice. It can be a decent value when circumstances are difficult financially.

That's it! The top protein sources for those on an income. There's no reason for not getting the protein your body requires every day to increase your fitness!

Chapter 8: Sample Meals

The best food choices to support the body building process can be a bit challenging. Once you've started eating as you should and begin to develop healthy eating habits, it'll become an aspect of your daily routine as a matter of course. A healthy diet is about making sure you are balancing different types of food and eating the right amount of what your body requires. Here's a list of nutritious foods that fit into the various categories that you should incorporate into your daily diet.

Proteins

Eggs

Soy

Turkey also known as chicken (White meat)

Shellfish

Steak or roast (Red meat)

Fresh fish

Tuna canned in a can

Tofu

Canned salmon

Complex Carbohydrates
Rice
Oatmeal
Legumes corn
Acorn squash
Yams
Potatoes
Sweet potatoes
Vegetables
All kinds that are water-based.
Green beans
Tomatoes
Asparagus
Spinach
Cabbage
Lettuce
Onions
Carrots
Peas
Mushrooms
Radish
Cauliflower
Leeks
Celery
Broccoli
Bok Choy

Zucchini Squash
Fruit
1 cup of grapes
1 cup berries
3 tiny Apricots
1 apple
1/4 melon
1 orange
1 mango
1 small papaya
1/2 grapefruit
1 banana
Dairy
1 cup of cottage cheese (low fat)
1 yogurt
1 cup of non-fat milk (You can also choose vanilla soy milk as an alternative)
Wheat Products
2 cups pasta
1 bagel
Whole wheat tortillas
2 slices of bread (whole wheat)
Snack Foods
Raw vegetables
Dried fruit
Plain popcorn

Nuts

Non-wheat cereals

Rice cakes

As we have mentioned the best diet has some of each type of foods. Thus, having a nutritional supplement to your diet is essential as detailed in a future section. In general, as we've mentioned previously it is recommended to eat five or six smaller meals throughout the day instead of cramming everything into three big meals. It is possible to schedule a meal every two or twice every 2 1/2 to 3 hours. For a start with, try a couple of the following dishes.

Meal 1

Have a treat with a vegetable breakfast that includes 1 whole egg with 3 egg whites as well as a cup of fresh vegetables. If you'd like to, you can include meat or chicken that is lean and healthy.

Meal 2

A protein shake, or a cup of yogurt

Meal 3

1 bagel

Small raw vegetable

6 8 ounces of chicken

Meal 4

3-4 ounces' of chicken

1-piece fruit

Meal 5

1 cup brown rice 1 cup brown

1 cup veggies (grilled)

6 ounces' fish

Meal 1

1 cup yogurt

1 banana

3 packs of instant oatmeal

1 cup cottage cheese

Meal 2

1 large baked potato

Protein shake

Meal 3

1 cup yogurt

8 ounces of chicken breast

1 apple

2 cups pasta

Meal 4

One or two cups of broccoli

1 can tuna

Meal 5

1 cup brown rice 1 cup brown

Protein shake

Meal 6

2 cups rice

1 cup vegetables

8 ounces of broiled fish

Meal 1

1 cup berries

Breakfast burrito that includes 1 egg, scrambled in whole and salsa, three egg whites as well as one cup of onions and green peppers.

1 cup cottage cheese

Meal 2

1 cup of raw vegetables

Protein shake

Meal 3

1 large potato. Cut thin slices, then brush it with olive oil, then bake them in the oven until they're crispy.

A salmon burger with onions that has been cooked in fry pans that are non-stick along with an egg white as well as canned salmon. Serve the burger in a breaded whole grain bun.

1 garden salad lightly drizzled by olive oil, red wine and vinegar.

Meal 4

1 cup yogurt

Protein shake

Meal 5

2 cups pasta

8 ounces of chicken breast. Cut it into smaller cubes, fry it in olive oil, then season with salt, garlic, oregano and basil.

1 cup of broccoli or cauliflower mix

I cup tomatoes, cooked

Meal 6

1 cup melon

Protein shake

1 cup yogurt

These menus are suggestions and you're able to alter the plans to suit what's best for you. It is always beneficial to plan your meals ahead of time. You can also prepare certain meals, for example, cutting your vegetables and placing them in the refrigerator , so you don't have to be working hard when it comes to meal time. The key is preparation the consistency of your meals.

Furthermore, you don't have to be precise in measuring the amount of food you are recommended to consume in meals. This kind of precision isn't necessary for novices! Simply a glance in accordance with the following chart should be sufficient:

PortionSize

1 ounce of meatMatchbox

3 ounces of meatDeck cards

8-ounce paperback meatThin book

3 ounces of fish Checkbook

1 ounce cheeseFour dice

1medium potatoComputer mouse

2tablespoon peanut butter 2 tablespoon Ping Pong ball

1 cup pastaTennis ball

1 bagel Hockey puck

To assist you cooking I've also put together several recipes that are worth trying within the following chapter.

COOKING TO BODY MASS

The great thing about healthy meals is that they don't need to be an experienced in the kitchen to prepare them. A nutritious meal is a great addition to your exercise routine and can help to ensure that you are getting the proper amount of proteins, carbohydrates and fats that are required for growth in your muscle. Cooking is also a great way to get to know your diet and figure out the exact ingredients you require in your meals. Be sure to ensure that your diet contains all the essential nutrients are essential for building muscle. Here are some recipes you can kick in your cooking process:

Cereal Casserole

8 oz. yogurt

Skimmed milk

Honey

Cereal

A bowl is used to mix the cereal according to the quantity you prefer.

Pour milk into bowl until it is higher than the cereal that is in the bowl.

Include yogurt, then add cereal as well as milk.

Serve the honey drizzled on top.

Protein Pancakes

Whole egg

11 egg whites

1 cup oatmeal

1-pack of jelly sugar free flavor

Within a bowl mix all the ingredients thoroughly.

On a non-stick pan, set to medium-high heat, pour over the contents in the bowl.

Tune patties or Salmon

1 whole egg

1 onion

One teaspoon parsley

1 can tuna or salmon (to your preference)

1 tablespoon salt

Three medium-sized potato, cooked and mashed

One teaspoon of pepper

A bowl is used to mix the potatoes, salt pepper onions, parsley and tuna.

Form the dough into patties.

Then fry these patties with olive oils until they turn brown.

Chicken Ole

One can of chili beans with a spicy kick.

1 onion cut into pieces

One can diced tomato

8 ounces of chicken breast chunked

Sauté the breast of chicken in olive oil and onions in a pan.

Add the tomatoes and chilli beans to the pan, and stir them well. Cook for about 10 minutes.

To enhance the flavor, sprinkle low-fat Cheddar cheese on the top.

Lightning Fast Fajitas

1 pound of steak in small pieces

3 . 3 cloves garlic

1 green pepper large with a slit cut in strips

1 red pepper that has been stripped

1 medium onion, stripped

1 teaspoon chili powder

Ground pepper

Lemon juice

In a skillet cook the garlic with the lemon juice (approximately 1 minute).

Add the beef along with the chilli powder to the fry pan until the beef has cooked to the desired level of degree of rareness. Add the peppers and onions.

Cook until the vegetables are tender. Turn up the heat until the veggies begin to brown.

Add the wheat tortillas, and mix thoroughly.

Chicken Cacciatore

28 ounces of can of crushed tomato

1 tablespoon chopped parsley

1/2 teaspoon oregano

3/4 teaspoon salt

2 lbs. chicken breast skinless and boneless

1/4 teaspoon of thyme

1 onion chopped

1 green pepper chopped

3 cloves of garlic, press

Cooking spray

Pepper to taste

The fry pan is coated with cooking spray, and then set it to medium-high temperature. Cook the chicken until it is it is cooked through. Set aside.

Cook onion until soft. Then add oreganoand tomato pieces, salt pepper parsley, thyme, and salt.

In the remaining 15 minutes, lower the temperature to low, and stir to the desired amount. Add your chicken, and then cover.

Cook for an additional 45 minutes.

The lid of the pan is removed and cook for about 15 minutes.

Consume brown rice over it.

Broiled Fish

14 ounces of diced tomatoes containing basil, garlic, oregano

1 lb. fish fillets

In a skillet, place the fish fillets on a line. Serve with tomatoes.

Cover the skillet with a lid and set it the heat to medium. Cook until the fish is cooked. It should take about 15 minutes. Consume plain or with brown rice.

Fish Dijon

1 clove of garlic, chopped and crushed

1 cup lemon juice

6 fillets of fish washed, pat dry and rinsed

2 tablespoons capers drained

1 1/2 lbs. zucchini, halved

2 tablespoons Dijon mustard

Paprika

Mix mustard and garlic in the bowl. Make a big pan and arrange the zucchini and fish in a row. Pour lemon juice over it and then over the upper rack cook for approximately five minutes. Flip the fish over and spread the garlic and mustard mixture on the fish.

Broil until the fish cooks and zucchini has turned brown.

Sprinkle capers and paprika on top.

Servings: 6

Stuffed Chicken

4 chicken breasts boneless and skinless

1 egg lightly beat

1 onion chopped

8 ounces ricotta cheese, low fat

1 package of dried and thawed frozen spinach

Salt and pepper

Cut the breasts of chicken in half. Then flatten them.

A bowl is used to mix eggs, cheese as well as spinach and onions. Place a part of the mixture inside each chicken breast.

By using butcher's string to tie the four breasts of a chicken. You could also place toothpicks instead.

Bake the breasts for approximately 35 minutes at 350°F. Serve hot.

Turkey Sauce

1 jar spaghetti sauce

1 cup portabella mushrooms, chopped

1 pound of ground beef or turkey

1 teaspoon allspice
1 onion chopped
Salt and pepper
1 teaspoon of red pepper flaked
Cook the meat in red pepper until golden.
Add mushrooms and chopped onion and add salt, pepper and allspice.
Add spaghetti sauce.
Eat over your favorite noodles.
Lemon as well as Pepper tuna
Seasoning for lemon pepper
One can of tuna
Spray cooking spray that is non-stick on the fry pan. Place tuna in the pan and sprinkle with the seasoning.
Cook until the dish is cooked according to your preference.
You can have it as is and with pasta.
It is also served cold, if desired.
Worcestershire Tuna
Worcestershire Sauce
One can of tuna
No-fat cheese
First, spray a zero calories cooking spray for non-stick on the fry pan.

Then, in the skillet mix the tuna and Worcestershire sauce, according to preference, and cook until it attains that desired consistency.

You may add cheese if desired. Switch off the heat and allow the cheese to melt.

Take a bite of plain bread, sprinkled over or with brown rice.

Rice, Chicken and Beans

1/4 can of red beans

1 cup of brown rice cooked

2 tablespoons barbeque sauce

Chicken breast, cooked , and shreds

Mix chicken, beans and rice in the form of a Tupperware or large bowl.

Pour the barbeque sauce into a bowl and mix until it's thoroughly coated. Serve.

Egg-Salad Sandwich

1/2 can tuna (optional)

2 slices of whole wheat bread

2 tablespoons low-fat mayonnaise

Spinach leaves, or lettuce shredded

1 cup yellow mustard

3-4 egg whites cooked in boiled eggs

Ground black pepper

Mix egg whites into the bowl of a large size. Add mustard, tuna, mayonnaise and black pepper.

Mix thoroughly and spread the mix over the bread. Put lettuce leaves or spinach on the bread on top, and then cover it with another slice of whole wheat bread.

Tuna Casserole

1 cup of canned peas washed and drain

2 tablespoon low-fat mayonnaise

1/2 cup cottage cheese

3-4 cups pasta, cooked

1/4 cup low-fat cheddar cheese, shredded

2 cans of tuna that has been drained

Black pepper

Combine all the ingredients in a bowl and mix it well. After serving, heat in the microwave for about a minute.

Chicken Deluxe

5 ounces of red potatoes

2 Tablespoons Cajun rub

Two teaspoons of cayenne pepper

8 ounces of chicken breast

1.5 cups of green beans frozen

Two teaspoons of jalapeno peppers crushed and dried

2 pinches salt

Tabasco sauce (you can substitute the other sauces for hotness)

A bowl is used to mix the chicken, cayenne pepper hot sauce, salt and cayenne pepper. Then, roll the chicken breasts in the rest of the ingredients and then store in the refrigerator for up to 10 hours.

A Foreman-style grill is ideal for this recipe.

Prepare the grill and place the chicken breasts on it. The chicken breast should cook for about 7.5 minutes.

Cut your red potato. Place the potatoes into the oven. Cook until soft. Then, take the potatoes out and then add the spinach. Microwave for a couple of minutes.

Mash the potatoes, and garnish by adding jalapeno and salt. Add salt in the rest of the beans.

Chicken Asparagus Rolls

2 slices turkey bacon, low-fat

1 chicken breast

1 tablespoon honey

2 asparagus sticks

1 teaspoon Dijon mustard

Salt and pepper as per your personal preference

Trim off the excess fat of the chicken breasts after washing it. Cut it into three slices. In a container, mix chicken with honey, mustard, salt and pepper. Set aside and let wait for approximately 25 minutes to marinate.

Clean the asparagus, cut off its hard ends and then take off the scales using the vegetable peeler. Place a piece of turkey bacon to each slice of chicken. Place the final asparagus stick and then roll.

Once you are sure that the Chicken Aspagarus Roll is ready to be served, tie the turkey bacon with two pricks of wood. Make sure you put the pricks in such an order to ensure that the chicken stays well-shaped.

Set the electric grill at 375 degrees, and cook the rolls for about seven minutes.

You can also bake them to 375°F for approximately 25 minutes.

Quick Scallops

Two cloves of minced garlic

1 pound of bay scallops washed

1 teaspoon of dried parsley

1/4 cup white wine that is dry and unpasteurized

Juice of 1 lemon

In a medium-sized fry pan, heat wine to medium heat. Add garlic and cook for about a minute. Then add lemon juice , and parsley. Cook the pan, covered, for 1 minute.

Then, add the scallops and cook them until they become opaque and not translucent.

Servings: 2-3

Roasted Vegetables

1 . A large clove cut into cloves, then peel off the skin.

6 peeled and cut shallots

6 peeled parsnips, quartered

1 teaspoon dried thyme

6 carrots peeled and cut in quarters

1 tablespoon dried rosemary

4 tablespoons olive oil

2 onions peeled, chopped into 6- 8 wedges

In Oven:

Set the oven to the setting of about 400 F.

Get a roasting dish and mix all the vegetables in it. Include salt as well as pepper according to your preference and then add oil. Stir to cover. Bake until the mixture is tender. This takes about 80 minutes.

On the Grill:

The grill should be set to medium-high temperatures. Use a tinfoil container, and then mix together all the vegetables. Include salt, pepper and as desired. Then add olive oil and mix until well the meat is coated. In the end, roast for approximately 30 minutes (until the meat is tender).

This recipe is great with meat, fish and even chicken.

Chicken-Salad Roll-ups

1/3 cup non-fat yogurt

2 tablespoons dried fruit pieces

1 pound boneless, uncooked chicken cooked

1/8 cup diced celery

2.25 tablespoons of sunflower seeds

A leaf of lettuce that is fresh

Cut the chicken in pieces and put it in the bowl of a mixer. Add yogurt, fruit pieces sunflower seeds, celery into the bowl.

Pick a leaf of lettuce then pour some mixture into the bowl over it, and then roll it upwards in a tight.

Continue to repeat the steps until the entire mix is used up.

Serve immediately.

If you intend to eat them later put them in plastic wrap correctly.

Servings: 2

The Foil is filled with fish

1 teaspoon of parsley

1 teaspoon fresh Dill

1/2 pound of halibut, cut into two pieces

1 carrot, julienne

One chopped, green onion

1 cup white wine Dry

4 small zucchini, julienne

1 tomato chopped

Ground pepper

Pre-heat the oven up to 400 F.

Divide the foil in two pieces, each measuring 12 inches and set the pieces of fish one on each square piece. Put a zucchini, carrot green onion, tomatoes on the fish piece. Sprinkle with pepper, herbs and wine.

Cut the ends of foil and secure by the foil. Cook the salmon for about 15 minutes.

Servings: 2

Mass Building Shake

1/2 cup of cranberry juice

1 cup of strawberries that have been frozen

1/4 cup egg whites

Half a banana

3/4 cup of soymilk, vanilla flavor

1 cup of ice cubes

Mix all the ingredients at a high temperature for approximately 30 seconds.

Energy Salad

3/4 cup sprouts

One cup of salad broken into smaller pieces

1/3 cup carrots that have been shredded

1 tablespoon olive oil 1 tablespoon olive

1/3 cup of mushrooms, cut into slices

1 cup sunflower seeds

1/3 tomato, sliced

2 tablespoons juice of a lemon

12 cucumbers, peeled and cut into slices

1/2 cup spinach chopped into bite-sized pieces

1/3 avocado, cubed

A dash made of parsley and thyme and basil

Blend the sprouts, spinach sunflower seeds, cucumber and mushrooms, as well as avocado, lettuce, tomato the carrots, spinach, and spinach inside a bowl for salad.

Blend lemon juice and olive oil and other herbs in a the screw-tight jar. Shake the mixture and then mix it thoroughly. Pour the mix over the salad.

Broccoli Salad

1 teaspoon of ground black pepper

1/4 cup non-fat yogurt

1/2 cup of sliced mushrooms

1 stalk of celery cut into pieces

1 Cup cooked and cooked broccoli chopped

1/2 pound steak cooked and cut into pieces

1/2 teaspoon mustard

1 head lettuce

1 tablespoon lemon juice

1 onion green, cut into slices

1/2 slice tomato

1 cup of cooked and cut green beans

1 tablespoon of red wine vinegar

Fresh parsley

Mix together the green beans, mushrooms, onion, steak, celery as well as broccoli into a big bowl of salad.

Use a screw-tight container. Mix vinegar, yogurt and mustard. Add pepper, mustard and lemon juice. Shake the mix until it's completely blended.

On the lettuce leaf, lay the salad out and then dress it with the mix. Add tomato and parsley slices.

Protein Smoothie

1 banana

1/3 cup blueberries that have been frozen

1 cup vanilla yogurt, fat free

1 cup milk, fat free

1/2 cup beaten egg

1/4 cup frozen cherries.

Add all ingredients to the blender. Blend until the mixture is smooth.

If you're looking to increase your body mass and strength, nutrition is something you shouldn't make a sacrifice to. It's not required to follow a strict diet, but you should be aware of what you are feeding your body and whether it is maximizing your workouts or not.

Another thing your body requires to get through a workout is a good night's rest.

Chapter 9: Bodybuilding Nutrition

Many personal trainers and bodybuilders will inform you that building muscle is more than fifty% nutrition. After working out, muscle growth and repair require lots of protein and nutrients that come from a balanced and healthy diet. It doesn't what you do, how much effort you train or how lucky you are in the genetics department. Without a balanced diet it's difficult to build strong and well-nourished muscles. The tips below on nutrition will assist you in building strong muscles.

Eat a lot of protein

Muscles are made up of proteins. To build muscles, it is recommended to consume between 1 and 1.5 grams of protein for every pound body weight per day. Certain individuals see greater results when they consume close to 2-grams of protein per kilogram body weight. This is especially true for those who are performing intense training regimens.

Don't Refrain from Carbs

The bodybuilding exercises require lots of energy. When compared to proteins and fats carbohydrates are the most readily available source of energy that your body uses. A significant portion of your daily caloric intake should be from carbohydrates. For strength training to be fueled it is essential to consume at two grams of carbs per pound body weight every day. It's a good idea to eat carbohydrates with each meal. Be sure to stay clear of sugary carbs and make sure that your carbohydrates starchy that are unprocessed, whole and unprocessed.

Remember Fats

It is suggested that 20-30% of your daily intake of calories is derived from fats. Fats play an important role within our bodies. For instance, fats are required for the synthesis and regulation of testosterone hormone. This hormone, as explained in chapter 1, is essential to build muscle mass.

Select red meats such as ground beef and steak for high-fat saturated oils (these are also protein-rich) mixed nuts avocados,

avocados and olive oil and peanut butter to get monounsaturated fats. You can also choose oily fish (trout or salmon, catfish, etc.) as well as flax seeds and walnuts to get the essential omega-3 fats.

Drink Smart Shakes

Instead of consuming daily with 4,000 calories of all-natural foods it is possible to make high-calorie shakes that provide your every day needs. Protein shakes are delicious and can be made with eggs, whey protein powder crushed almonds, oatmeal, ground coconut and flax seeds, and nutseed butters.

Eat frequently

Since your metabolism rises after exercising it is possible that you need to take a snack every 2 or 4 hours.

Nutrition for Pre and Post Workouts

If you're hoping to take advantage of each training session What you feed your body prior to and following training sessions is important. Carbohydrates, your body's primary fuel source, as well as proteins, which are the main components of muscle mass should be consumed quickly prior to and following the workout. A shake of protein that contains the protein powder whey is a great option during this period since it contains both carbohydrates and proteins. After and before exercising, stay away from eating fats that are difficult to digest.

Eat before you go to bed

As you rest your body goes into an in-built repair mechanism where muscles get repaired, and proteins are created. Prior to bed, consume shakes and snacks that have the slow-digesting protein casin to help to promote muscle growth

Chapter 10: Different Types Of

Sarms

Because SARMS are relatively new to the marketplace there are various forms and types of SARMS are available. Below are the most popular SARMS available today and most appropriate for fitness, bodybuilders and fans:

Ostarine MK-2866

A kind of SARM is known as Ostarine MK-2866. It is generally prescribed to avoid and treatment of muscle weakness. These health issues may be genetic in nature due to HIV/AIDS, or other ailments. There are studies in places that suggest that the medication could soon be suggested as a part the hormone replacement treatment (HRT).

SARMS create anabolic selective activity in a variety of androgen receptors. There isn't any androgenic action however , for non-skeletal muscle tissues as it is when you use testosterone or anabolic steroids.

The use of Ostarine MK-2866 may help by gaining strength and muscle mass.

How Ostarine MK-2866 Functions

The use of SARMS allows more protein be integrated to ensure that muscle tissue can grow. The use of Ostarine MK-2866 is directly dependent on the results that a person can achieve taking various types of steroids. But, they are able to use them without threatening other sexual organs like the prostate.

If this SARM is taken it can cause anabolic results for the muscles. It's a novel treatment for health issues, such as AIDS as well as cancer. It is widely utilized by bodybuilders and athletes to offer their bodies greater strength and muscles. It's also employed to aid in the recovery process following surgery or injuries. A lot of athletes take a moderate dose of 15 mg every day to lessen the risk of sustaining an injury. The development of joints can be seen within the span of a week.

In the event that Ostarine MK-2866 Utilized

There are a variety of cycles that one could choose to use Ostarine MK 2866 for. One of them is a bulking one where they want to build muscles that are lean. This provides them with the chance to gain weight which is predominantly muscle. This weight gain could be as high as 7 pounds. They can be observed over eight weeks when you consume 25 mg daily. The daily dose should not need exceed 40 mg daily. For optimal results, it has to be taken every day.

In a process of reducing body fat, also known as cutting, reducing calories and increasing workout duration can help you build more muscles. Cutting without the use of SARMS can result in the loss of the muscle mass, which is irritating. This happens because of a decrease in hormone levels and slowing of the metabolism. When you take Ostarine MK-2866 in the treatment of weakening or loss of muscle won't need to be a worry any longer. To cut a cycle, the dosage is 15 mg daily is consumed over a period of between 6 and 8 weeks.

The nutritional benefits that this SARM provides is very encouraging. The ability to efficiently lose weight and keep the growth in muscle is extremely beneficial. Utilizing steroids, you take a longer time to experience the effects however this is not the case with Ostarine MK 2866. It is also not a risk for liver damage. damaged, which is a typical adverse effect of using steroids. Also, it won't cause issues with blood pressure.

Benefits from Ostarine MK-2866 over Steroids

There are many benefits to using Ostarine MK-2866 in place of steroids. Below are the most unique benefits worth noticing:

*Not too harsh on the liver.

*Less expensive

*Won't alter blood pressure

*Can help prevent issues with joints and bones due to injuries

Effects are visible immediately.

There is no chance of water retention.

There is no risk of estrogen-related adverse negative effects

*Provides nutritional benefits when cutting calories

LGD-4033

Another kind of Selective Androgen Receptor Modulator is known as LGD-4033. LGD-4033 can be described as an oral device that is not steroidal, however it may provide many of the same advantages as anabolic steroids. The medical use of LGD-4033 is to treat muscle weakening. This could be the result of problems with cancer or loss of muscle due to the natural ageing process.

The same advantages as testosterone are offered by LGD-4033. The distinction is that the individual using LGD-4033 isn't concerned about potential negative side negative effects. When you take testosterone, there may be the risk that the body isn't responding well, or even creating a potential for the liver. Although this drug is taken orally, it's not toxic to the liver.

LGD-4033 is among the most well-known SARMS utilized due to its potency. But it also feels calming for the body when compared with the use of steroids. If you're looking for benefits but not all the issues, this may be the solution they've been looking for.

What is LGD-4033?

LGD-4033 functions by enlarging the androgen receptors, selectively. Anabolic effects on muscles and bones occur rather than negatively altering the prostate or glands, which could be caused through the use of steroids. LGD-4033 has recently been engaged in a study with volunteers called Phase 1 Multiple Ascending Dose. It was random, double blind testing phase in which placebo was used. The aim was to verify that the usage of LGD-4033 is safe and easy to use with a dosage not exceeding 22 mg daily.

How to use LGD-4033?

For many bodybuilders and athletes LGD-4033 is used as a bulking phase, to provide the body with lean mass and reduce body fat. LGD-4033 use can also boost total strength, which allows an individual the ability to tackle more challenging training sessions. If LGD-4033 is used to bulk up, a healthy diet high in protein is crucial. A higher intake of calories could be necessary in the event that the person who is using the product is expected to bulk up by 10 pounds or more than the recommended amount. The recommended dosage is between 5 and 10 mg daily, for 8 weeks.

To cut a cycle It might be beneficial to utilize LGD-4033 along with other SARMS, including S-4 and the GW-501516. This is referred to as the SARMS Triple stack. Its purpose is to build an extra amount of mass while also cutting fat. The recommended dosage for this kind of cycle is between 3 and 5 mg daily, for a time period of 8 weeks.

Risk Factors for LGD-4033

The findings of various studies reveal that there is little chance of adverse effects of LGD-4033 use. This is good news for those who want to build muscles and lose weight without resorting to steroids that can cause dangerous side effects that are associated to their use. In addition, the fact SARMS aren't harmful for the liver an additional reason to think about having them instead of steroids. They're also priced reasonably and so everyone can take them in without stressing about cost.

GW-501516

A PPAR modulator provides the body with the chance to utilize more glucose and build additional muscle tissue. The GW-501516 molecule is one of the PPARs. It might be referred to as GSK-516 or GW1516 too. It is a great aid in reducing or even reverse many issues in males who are overweight or suffer from pre-diabetes due to issues in their metabolism. It is an effective treatment to cut the weight gain and other diseases that can be linked to it.

How does GW-501516 Work?

The GW-501516 drug is an agonist that is selective and has high affinity, and is extremely efficient. Numerous studies on the PPAR receptor in laboratory rats show that it regulates various proteins used by the body to generate energy. Rats who had low metabolism and excess fat were treated with the GW-501516 drug and could lose weight while also boosting energy levels overall.

When to Utilize GW-501516?

The primary reason for GW-501516 use is to help improve levels of survival. However professional athletes cannot utilize GW-501516 as it falls into the category of prohibited substances. This means that athletes don't have an unfair advantage over their competitors. If you are looking for ways to speedily improve the quality of life, this product could aid in providing quick results. The recommended dosage for GW-501516 is 10 mg daily.

Another common use of GW-501516 is to reduce body fat. The fat will begin to fall off quickly and isn't catabolic. Losing fat won't cause muscle loss as well, which is the main benefit that users of the GW-501516 like. It's a good idea to use it for fat loss along alongside Ostarine and S4 which are both SARMS to ensure that loss of muscle is only small. The recommended dosage for the GW-501516 dosage is 10 mg per day, but many people take as high as 20 mg per day in order to lose as the body fat they are able to in the 8-week cycle.

Potential Risks associated with the GW-501516

There are a few reports about the possible side effects and risks associated with the use of the GW-501516 drug. Certain reports about laboratory rats indicate that it may cause cancer. In other studies it is concluded that there aren't enough data to support or disprove this assertion. The fact that it's not harmful to the liver is important to stress. Because GW-501516 is fast-acting and is less expensive than steroids and is an extremely popular option.

Chapter 11: The Philosophy Section

More Than Your Gladiator Body

There's an explanation for why Spartans and gladiators, as well as warriors from the past could easily be feared as monsters. For them, their training were their life. They were required to fight or to die. They didn't hesitate about it. Even if you're struggling to maintain motivation levels and the discipline needed to drive to the car and drive to Gold's Gym for them, it wasn't an issue. You can do it or you'll be dead it's that easy.

It's not to say that they were the social pillars. A man who was fashioned out of training pits that only is able to crush people is reminiscent of "The Mountains" of Game of Thrones; a killer machine that was later utilized as a pawn in intelligent powers.

Nowadays, you don't need to worry about this happening (in the majority of countries anyway) however, in the beginning of this book, I have been criticized for declaring that I'd trade my large muscles in exchange for Bill Gates' big brain power.

And I believe in this assertion. It is essential to have both regular and emotional intelligence to succeed in life. This "clobbering soldier" archetype exists in the present. It's my friends who I work with or even a lot of the guys I've met within the U.S. military. They're massive, they're strong and they're skilled, they're killers however, certain of them with all respect can't locate Spain on the map, they consider that Saddam Hussein caused 9/11, and aren't sure how to interact with people they've never met at a party or nightclub.

It's not going to work at ALL. If you're lacking on these fronts, then I strongly recommend you to set the weights on for a few weeks and work on the rest of who you are.

It is important to see yourself as an ARMY PHILOSOPHER. This is the most powerful perspective a man can possess.

I believe that the men I've mentioned earlier could be warrior philosophers, and be educated, knowledgeable of the world, aware of the past and important events and also have the social graces to woo business partners and attract women by using their tongues and not just abs. But they don't invest any effort in these things. Just like ignoring the gym, their abilities diminish. They believe that they can get all their weaknesses solved by going to fitness, however they're in the wrong.

Similar to that "clobbering character of warrior" I've just mentioned the big buffoon is usually targeted by clever criminals. They'll tell you "go beat that guy" as well as "go shoot them" and they don't have the self-awareness necessary to question their orders or take to take care.

Again I'm not convinced that this is the case in the world of the beginning in the literal sense. But, in certain ways it could occur if you do not develop your brain and become smart. Being uninformed means that you'll end up being a tough badass that is doing in a very shady job and doesn't know how to get himself out of the situation, since more intelligent people manipulate and exploit the man constantly.

No one wants to be used And "goons" tend to be the ones who are always targeted by the criminals. Don't let that happen to you.

Words of Discipline

If you're developing your Mind or your BODY both require discipline. There's been plenty of articles written on becoming more disciplined. The issue is that your particular situation is different. But, there are at least two things that I have learned from and I'm certain they can assist you.

The main reason that people do not use your gym subscriptions that they experience a sudden, fleeting motivation. They decide, for instance, around new Years, "This will be the year" and they sign up for a membership, in February and then they're out of it.

The first thing you need to do is identify two different aspects: short-term motivation as well as an entirely new way of thinking. The first is when you are experiencing specific emotions at that exact moment in time. These emotions will eventually fade as your mood shifts. A philosophical view however, means the essence of your being has changed into something entirely new.

Consider your current beliefs. One of them is that you should take good care for your dental health. That's why you brush your teeth daily. There is nothing that can stop you from doing it, because it's etched into your brain, and most likely, it was your parent's task to take care of that. You also had to visit the dentist early on and have your teeth drilled, or a root canal procedure done, so you're surrounded by that negative reaction that stops you from breaking free of the ethos.

What is the philosophy behind giving back to the community? I hope you've got that one. You're kind to your aunts, cousins and parents. You wave and smile at the waiters. You want people around you to feel happy because you too would like to feel great and contribute to making the world a better. Alternative is to wander around acting like a slob. Maybe you've been like this in college or high school and then discovered how hard it is to be a bad person. It leads to broken relationships, dismal relationships and a life that was miserable because you did not treat people well. So your philosophy changed.

So , how do I change my stance on working out?

In the beginning, you must to be aware of your priorities.

I'd like to make it crystal clear (and I've had to deal with many gym snobs that believe that this isn't true) there is no need for a physique builder in order to be healthy. You should exercise every day to improve your heart health. Cut out the bad grains, sodas and processed sugary drinks. Learn ways to manage stress. Buy organic. Have a test with a doctor. Follow these steps and you stand a high likelihood of living to the upper 80s or 90s (thin as an old post all the time and lacking muscles) or even dying with your marbles intact, able to live a full the rest of your life until you reach you get old or a tumor gets to you.

On the other hand, you could be a bodybuilder who is struck with a cancer lightning bolt at some point, and is dead within 5 weeks. The body is swollen at the end and look like a Holocaust victim, despite the amount of work you've put into building yourself up.

However, the same thing could occur to the man who is living a very well-balanced life.

In the meantime, a few assholes drink Coca Cola every day, chain smokers, is obese and constantly stressed. He lives to 105and is miserable all the way and yet 'healthy'.

There's a lot of wackiness associated with our bodies and in the process of dying. It's not always easy to predict and you'll never be completely in control. There is also the possibility of randomness.

Have I made you feel depressed yet? Good. It's becoming a pain. Continue looking.

The positive side is there's things you can take control of. One is the way you spend your time in the days you've been granted. Another thing that you control can be your legacy.

Imagine that people are thinking of your future. They'll think "Yeah, Steve. The guy who inspired you was Steve. He was sculpted as Apollo, the God of Apollo. When I was with him made me feel more secure because of the way his appearance and how he carried himself and his manner of speaking that was always the sun shining through. He was the type that I would want my children to be."

There's a chance that you have many of these traits even if you're not as thin in the post. But how much of an impact can you really make by being a slack guy? You'll remain loved and live an enjoyable life, but you'll never be the hot DYNAMITE you could be.

The most epic thing happens the moment when a skinny man becomes gorgeous, chiseled man. Then, he is regarded as God among men.

In the wake of telling those things to you, now imagine that you're in your final days, and you're thinking of this stupid Kindle book that you read years ago (back when people didn't have Kindles as well and it was not an apocalyptic wasteland) and you're thinking "Wow I could have been DYNAMITE, an source of inspiration for others around me, gorgeous sexually attractive, hot and tough Imagine the various experiences I might have had should I have chosen this path for myself and did not. My life was great however, I could've made it really exciting, and also. What's the reason I didn't simply take one simple year of my time to devote to it?" Wow, that's pretty hardcore.

Imagine yourself in the shoes of those. Imagine this is you. If this has an impact on you that is profound emotional response If it does, then I've got good news for you. It means that your mindset has changed. It'll soon be simple to get in your vehicle and head into the gymnasium. In fact , you'll be nervous if you're unable to do it as you would when you didn't brush your teeth at night.

However, life is meaningless. I might just get a terminal illness and die

It's amazing how much negativity can be for us. Perhaps you felt depressed when I wrote the piece about the possibility of ending in a cancerous state and appear like a victim of the Holocaust in the final days of your days regardless of how hard you tried.

Nihilism really is based on death and the philosophical premise that we will never exist therefore, we should forget about the present since we're all going to "the vacuum".

There's no reason to support all of these assertions. The universe and life are constantly evolving and changing. The fact that you will die isn't too bad as it's an opportunity to improvement. You must rely on others to make amends for the mistakes of your past and, when your body is aging you'll develop humility quickly. There's no reason to feel negative about anything, including this one.

For the death itself. Let me have a break. There will always be consciousness throughout the universe or otherwise, the universe wouldn't exist. When you finally start to croak, you'll either find YOUSELF in a new form , thinking "Damn it was quite an adventure and what's coming next?" or you will become something completely different and in a new form and body you'll eventually master (and your desire to learn it will be carried across the cosmos).

This will make you an immortal warrior, mastering each new creation that the universe can throw at you for all time. This may sound like abstract philosophical ideas however what I'm saying is factual.

Chapter 12: Exercise Plans

The first step in a weight training exercise regimen requires a degree of commitment. If you are beginning, you'll be able to exercise more often than the muscle heads that you have created. The reason for this is simple As you become more familiar, you get a better understanding of how you can make your muscles stronger and do more devious things that gives you more chances for recovery from. Children, naturally suffer from soreness and then bounce back faster because the arm that is solid isn't as authentic.

If "hurt" affects you, and causes your ability to draw back do not pressurize. It's ideal for athletes to suffer limited muscle injuries because it forces the body back and causes it to increase the amount of compensation (grow) in a certain extent in preparation for future tasks.

That's what bodybuilding is all about - the steady cycle of one step back, two walks forward, repeated seven days following week's start.

The practice setup is based on one participant in your body every day during your workout, and midweek, as well as the end of the week being your days off.

This is only an idea. You are able to alter it unexpectedly to meet your needs and locations.

In any exercise there is a need to first of all warm-up exercises. It could be as simple as stretching as you set your body for working. A warm-up before exercise can't only assist in getting your body ready to work out, but your mind will become organised too.

In the same way, you should take a suitable time to rest following your work out. This will reduce the likelihood of muscle soreness that is not cured and can help manage the level of adrenaline growing in your body as a consequence of your exercise. It could also be a fundamental expanding exercises as well as important unwinding.

In the end, it's important to begin with a straight line and not push yourself beyond the purpose of your imprisonment.

Make sure you choose weights that aren't overly important for you, however, they should give you enough security to build your muscles.

You can build a powerful amount of weight that you lift as you become more stable.

Day 1 - Upper Body

For going exercises, start by playing two games of 10-12 reps each.

Dumbbell press

Military press with a standing barbell

Pressing the triceps in a tense way

Side sidelong raise

Priests turn

Conort dumbbells in an arrangement

Dumbbell lines

Dumbbell shrugs

In the event that you encounter machines for weight, include the information to your action plan:

Pec deck butterflies

Pushdowns with V-bars

Lat pulls using an automatic pulley

Day 2 Day 2 - Abs and Lower Body

Start each step with two rounds of exercise of 10-12 reps on each side of the crunches, which can be done in a similar amount of reps from what you'll need.

Barbell squat

One leg barbell squat

Hops

Pressing the calf in a standing position

Strong leg barbell

Crunches

They can be particularly helpful in working out in your lower body. Here are some to think about today:

Leg pushes onto the machine that stacks plates

Leg extension machine

Hamstring turns that are arranged

Hamstrings that are in the hamstrings of a standing person turn

Stomach muscle machine

Day 3 - Relax

Day 4 - Upper Body

Make sure you're with 10-12 reps per set.

Make sure you catch up (get assistance if needed)

A arranged dumbbell that pound turns

Dumbbell presses against an inclined seat

Military press with a standing barbell

Standing bicep twists

Barbell tricep expansion

Upright barbell push

Front dumbbell raise

The equipment you'll be able to use for this day are:

Lines of connection that are arranged

Upright connection lines

Connection half breed of flies

Pushdowns of the triceps

Day 5 - Abs and Lower Body

Return to just two games of 10-12 reps each, along with the crunches that you can perform unlimited amounts of.

Pressing the calf in a standing position

Sways

Barbell squat

Solidified leg barbell

Standing calf raises

Crunches

The machine rehearses includes:

Leg pushes onto an stacked plate machine
Hamstring turns that are arranged
The bowing hamstring twists
Week's end to rest
If a multi-day training arrangement is not feasible for you, think about starting with a multi-day plan.

Be aware that it isn't going to happen in the same speed with a shorter time-intensive workout, but however should you begin slowly, it could be a game-changing event.

Here's an example of work-outs that span multiple days.

Day 1 Day 1 - Back, Chest and Abs

Complete three sets comprising 12-15 reps per course.

Constrained around push of barbell

Solidified deadlift for barbells with legged legs

Barbell situate press

Slant dumbbell press

Dumbbell flies

Crunches

Day 2 Day 2 Legs and Shoulders

Complete three sets that each comprise 12-15 reps.

Barbell squat

Calf raises arranged in a row

Front dumbbell raise

Side sidelong raise

Upright barbell push

Bounces

Barbell squats

Day 3 Day 3 Biceps, Triceps, and Abs

Complete three different courses consisting of 12-15 reps for each

Barbell bend

Slant dumbbell contort

Pressing the triceps in a tense way

Barbell triceps enlargement

Front dumbbell raise

The dumbbell's pound turns

Crunches

A half hour before your workout, it is recommended to consume some sugars and protein. This will ensure that you have the necessary energy to endure your entire workout.

When you do this, you're placing your body in an anabolic state that will allow you to gain the vitality and capability to effectively train your muscles.

While getting ready, there's an extensive circulation system for the muscles. If you consume carbohydrates and protein prior to an exercise, your body could make use of that circulatory system to exercise the muscles to their fullest.

Many people opt for an protein shake and rice in a bowl however, being that as it happens you may pick whatever foods you need to have the things you need.

It's a smart idea to monitor your workouts and the amount of reps and sets you're performing. Keep it on a scratch pad and, if you are able to increase the amount of sets and more reps, make it the effort to observe how long you took to reach that stage. Additionally, record the amount of weight you are able to lift and also when you will be able to create the weight.

It's also a good idea to start your first set without weight. This helps to initiate the muscle structure through the muscles. In the second set, add a bit of weight and repeat the exercise time.

If you think it's not enough basic, you can try adding weight. The objective is to increase weight until it's hard to complete 8-12 repetitions.

Remember, you need to create your body stronger, not lift weights.

Be sure to rest between sets to allow your body to transform and recuperate. It is usually one minute or two.

Be as active as you can without having to stop for more than one minute or even close to it otherwise your muscles will be nippy and all of the work you've done will be in vain.

It's a smart idea to mix in an exercise routine to keep your blood flowing. This could be a brief duration on a treadmill, or a walk.

The cardio can be beneficial for your body and will be paying attention to the most fundamental muscle the heart!

Amazing food is an essential part of a well-rounded fitness program for any designer.

Chapter 13: Bodybuilding

Reduce the bench gradually to the point that it almost touches your temple. Then, push the bench back up with an arc of sluggish, smooth motion. On the floor, fix your joints completely.

Don't sloop down on the cushion, sit as straight as you can.

If your muscle tissues are able to support some weight, the total strength of the muscle mass will increase slowly.

Many people describe lifting weights as toughness training. While they're not identical but they're both similar to one another.

In the following section I'll break down the most common exercises and exercise areas to make sure you be aware of exactly what they do and the muscle tissue group they focus on.

Exercises for Education.

Side Lateral Pinhead Raising.

By using a shoulder-sized hold take the bar in both hands. It is important to use the muscles to lift your weight. Not using energy.

This exercise can be done with pinheads or on a bench.

The key to this exercise is keeping those arms within a fixed place.

A lot of training centers offer the services of a personal fitness instructor, which includes the price of a subscription.

Then, press the bar until it is at an arm's length over your head.

Place yourself at the bottom of the bench and then place something like a business cushion or a few cushions in your lap. Place the crinkle bar into your hands, with your hands facing upwards.

Existing Tricep Press.

Body building is the process of forming muscle tissue fibers through various methods. It is achieved by muscle conditioning and weightlifting, a higher calories consumed and also being in a position to sit your body as it repairs itself and heals itselfbefore starting your exercise routine again.

It's also possible to do it by using pinheads or only one arm at the same time.

Here are a few of the more well-known examples:.

The specific combination of collections, representatives and workouts as well as weight is contingent upon the requirements of the body builder. Collections with fewer representatives may be completed with greater weights but have an less impact on endurance.

This exercise is best done with a unique preacher crinkle bench but you could also do it without it , with just a small change.

Place yourself on the back of a regular bench, with the pinheads resting upon your knees. Through a single, smooth movement move your body into your back and bring the pinheads towards an outdoor position and then above your shoulders. Your hands should be dealing with the forwards.

Another form of exercise that is weightlifting is resistance training.

Keep your arms straight and lift the weights up and around your sides until they're a bit above your shoulder.

Arms in the Stand force Press.

It uses the force of gravity to counteract the pressure generated by muscle mass through contraction. Weightlifting employs various tools specifically designed to target specific muscles and movements. Your arm joints should be bent at 90 degrees, keeping your arms parallel to the floor. Lift the weights over your breasts in triangular movements until they are in line with the body's center.

Follow the exact route downwards.

Keep your hands turned downwards while you raise the pinheads so that your shoulders in addition to your arms accomplish the work.

Resistance training is the practice of the use of hydraulic or flexible resistance to tighten instead gravity.

The focus of this area is on bodybuilding exercises using weights for contractors. Weightlifting increases the strength of your muscles as well as the size of the skeletal muscle mass.

Training is designed to focus on specific muscular tissue classes or groups, and food items are consumed in order to build the body's metabolic system and increase overall mass.

Equipment used for weightlifting comprises of pinheads, weights, pulley blocks, and stacks of weight using devices for weight or your body's own weight in push-ups, and chin-ups. Different weights can offer different types of resistance.

This includes adjusting the variety of collection, reps of workouts, speed as well as weight shifting to cause desired increases in endurance, stamina size, or form.

Be sure to raise the pinheads upwards as opposed to turning them down. Be sure not to lean backwards when doing this or you chance of injury to your back.

Relax your back to ensure that your head's top is in line with the bottom of the bench. When you're back, extend your arms above your head until the bar is directly in front of your eyes.

Standing straight, your feet spread apart, and your arms by your side. Keep a pinhead in each hand while your hands are moved toward your body.

Limit your elbow joints and keep your arms firmly in place during your workout.

Secure your legs as well as hips and keep your elbow joints small space beneath the bar. Make sure you press the bar until your arm is size above your head.

If you're new in weightlifting, do not "hop into it". You must build your endurance and exercising too much on your muscles could result in more injuries than to a good.

The instructors may suggest certain exercises to begin with, but the guidelines in this guide will definitely help you develop an exercise that is effective quickly and easily.

By using a shoulder-sized grip to grasp the bar, you must be able to hold it in both hands. It is important to use your muscles to lift the bar, and not using energy.

The weightlifting principles that are commonly used are very similar to the ones used in stamina training.

It is also about exercises that are performed with correct muscle mass groups and not transferring the weight across parts of the body in order to lift great weight.

Sit on a bench, holding a crinkle bar using an overhand grip. Remain in a reclining position to ensure that your head's top is not impacted by the bench. When you're seated back, extend the arms to your head and make sure the you are able to see straight across your eyes.

Some of your muscle tissues might be stronger than other muscles. The gradual growth of muscle mass allows it to develop a superior toughness over each other.

The focus of training for toughness is to increase muscular toughness and dimensions. Weightlifting is one type of strength training that makes use of weights to provide the primary force to build muscular tissue mass.

As you increase the weight, concentrate on keeping the weights balanced and in control.

If you don't utilize safe weightlifting techniques you are at chance of injury to your muscles that could hinder the general growth of your body.

Let's examine a handful of of the most popular exercises and programs in order that you can better understand the numerous strategies used in the weightlifting industry and general physical fitness.

Preacher Swirls.

Make the bench sit close to your chin and keep in mind that resistance is the strongest at the initial phase of the lift. The bar is gradually lowered, working muscles as you go down.

Reduce the bell to your upper chest or your chin based on which is more comfortable for you.

Pinhead Bench Press.

Gradually reduce them to your side.

Sitting Pinhead Swirl

Keep your back straight, and keep your head straight. Begin by placing the pinheads on your the size of your arms, with your hands in.

Place your arms on your top and then slowly reduce the weight.

Don't open the pinheads down. Reduce them while you work those muscles mass! You can perform this while standing, but the sitting position stops the bad type of exercise.

One-Arm Pinhead Row

Lean forward to make sure that you're supporting an entire weight on your upper body, with your left hand not working. Your back should be at a level and nearly identical to the floor.

Before beginning, focus ahead instead of to the floor so that you can keep your back straight. Make sure you tighten your abdominal muscles to prevent your body away from the side while you lift the pinhead.

Once you've taken the pinhead to the height you were looking for, you can gradually lower it back to the initial position. Transfer arms following one set.

Start with your right foot on the floor as well as your left knee resting on a bench.

Make sure to sit the ground and take a pinhead from your right-hander. The left arm must be secured to the joint in order that it can support all the load of your upper body.

Make sure you draw your elbow joint so that it can be. The pinhead must end approximately the same size as the upper part of your body.

Pinhead Shrugs

Place your feet directly at shoulder height. Take 2 pinheads and hold them with your arms and place them by your sides.

Sagging your shoulders to the extent that is possible. Then raise your shoulders upwards as you can so the same position, and gradually return to your starting point. It is also possible to rotate your shoulders by circling from the front to the back, and then pull back one more. This can also be accomplished with a weight.

Standing Calf bone Height Increases

This can be completed by using a specific device in a facility for training or altered to allow for use without the device. You must stand on the wall by putting your body in contact with the wall's surface, and your hands firmly on the wall and your feet on the floor.

Make sure your body is straight and slowly lift your heels until they are positioned on the tips of your feet. Keep the tightening for a few seconds then slowly return to your starting position, keeping your feet flat on the floor.

Crunches

Always lower as far as you can using your lower back.

Lay on your back, with your feet firmly on the floor, or sitting on a bench with your knees bent at 90 degrees. If you're laying with your legs on the bench put them about 3-4 inches apart and place your feet inwards so that they are in contact.

Then, press the little of your back into the floor to break the muscles of your stomach. Then, begin to lift your shoulders off of the floor.

Your shoulders need to be from the floor just about 4 inches. Likewise, your lower back must remain in the floor. Focus on slow, controlled exercise - don't cheat yourself by using energy!

Pinhead Hammer Curls

With a pinhead on each hand, you stand with your arms up to your sides. Make sure that your you'll also be able to see your hands interacting with one another. Make sure your arm joints are secured to your sides. Your upper body as well as joints must be in the exact position throughout the entire lift.

Keep your hands in contact with one another, and crinkle the right-hand man to your left shoulder. The arms should be pressed hard over the top of the raise before gradually reducing.

Do not change your wrists while lifting! You can also do one arm at a time or alternate.

Slope Pinhead Press

The weights should be pushed back towards a certain amount over your breasts, using your hands to work ahead.

Lower the weights slowly. Inhale while you reduce the weights, and exhale as you lift.

At each time, raise the shoulders to a shoulder level while pushing your back and shoulders hard against the bench.

Stay on the opposite side of a slope bench , which is evaluated in terms of the 45-degree angle. Take a pinhead with each hand, and place them on your upper legs.

Weights Squat

Keep your back straight as you can and keep your chin upwards, bend your knees, and slowly lower your hips downwards until your legs are parallel to the floor. Once you've gotten back to your lower position then push the weight upwards until you return to your starting position.

Set a weight on top on your back. Do not rest it against on your neck. Make sure you secure the bench using your hands approximately twice the size of your shoulder to each other.

Your feet should be placed shoulder width apart, and your toes need to be pointed only a small amount to the exterior, while your knees are in a straight line.

Do not lean back or curve your back to the side! You can use belts to help reduce the chance of a back injuries.

Upright Weights Row

Sit up straight and comprehend that you are holding weights about shoulder length apart. Pull the bar straight upwards towards your chin while keeping it in place with your body.

You should concentrate on drawing using your catches or your shoulder's front depending on what exactly you want to do the best. Then gradually reduce the intensity to the initial position.

Front Pinhead Raising

Bring the weight in your left hand and place it in the direction of your body in a broad arc until it's a little above the level of your shoulder.

Do not cut off by closing or leaning in the reverse! The lift could also be completed with two pinheads in the exact simultaneously or weights.

Make sure you have a pinhead in each hand, with the hands working the opposite direction. Your feet should be the same size as your shoulders to each other. Make sure to keep a slight bent elbow joint during your workout to ensure the arms remain straight but not securely.

In a controlled, fluid process, you can reduce the weight simultaneously lifting the weight of your right-hand hand, so that both arms are in motion at the simultaneously.

Rigid Leg Weights

Retract your steps gradually until you reach the highest position. It is possible to finish by knees slightly bent.

Put a few weights onto your back. Keep your head straight and also your back straight.

Bend your midsection and bend with your legs secure, and your upper body is parallel to the floor.

One Leg Squat Weights

Keep your head and neck to the upper body so that you're facing forward. Your shoulders must be straight and over your front foot.

Keep your back straight and raise your head. The tiny part of your back to the flooring to divide the muscles in your stomach. Bring the weights towards a point over your upper breasts using your hands to work ahead. You could use belts to help reduce the chance of a back injuries. Make sure your back is kept in check and your breast out during the entire training.

Keep your front foot level on the floor, place on your backs with hips (like you're preparing to relax in the chair) then extend the leg (of the front of your leg) and then move your body forward a bit towards the waistline.

Use a 12 - to 18-inch box or bench to perform this exercise. The bigger boxes, the more difficult the exercise. Set a weight behind your head, at the neck's base. Learn to comprehend the weights using both hands using a larger than the shoulder size grip.

Now, starting by your head, and then your upper body, lift yourself with your shoulders a bit forward and then upwards towards the ceiling and making sure your leg is aligned. Revert to the original place.

If you're having trouble cutting down on your own this much, you can reduce it by yourself until the front of your leg bent 90 degrees.

Maintain your foot at a at a level with the floor and take into consideration your toes in the future. Make sure you stand straight. Keep your back as tight and your chest out for the duration of your workout.

Your knee has to be straight across your toe. Your hips should be free of tension and your upper body should be straight across the middle of your leg.

Your body is reduced by regulating your body to the point that your lower foot (of your front foot) is in line with the ground.

In this moment the shoulders should be straight and your feet should be in front of you.

Take a stand about 2 or 3 feet away from the box and shift to ensure your box lies in front of you. Move one foot back and place your toes over the boxes.

Lunges

Then, gradually flex your knees. reduce your hips to the point that your back knee is removed from the floor. Pause briefly at this point, and after which you slowly align your legs, and then raise your body to a standing posture.

A complete set of reps and then switch legs, and repeat or switch legs after each repetition.

Set up a weight on your back top. Bring your breasts up and look directly ahead. Set your leg in the right direction with a long stride.

Make sure your knee doesn't go over your toes while in the down position! This can also be done by using pinheads on each hand instead of making use of weights.

Your foot should be a good distance ahead of you so that, when you bend the right leg, both your leg as well as your lower leg form an ideal angle.

Expansion of Triceps and Weights

Use your hands to hold a weight just a bit closer to each other in comparison to the size of your shoulder. Place your body on a bench with a slope and then set your head up on top.

Bar expenses are based on the size of your arm. Reduced bench in semicircular movement in front of your head until your arms are lower than your arms.

Keep your arms in close proximity to your head. Return to the starting position. It could be completed using a straight bar, two pinheads, standing or sitting or using 2 pinheads, as well as your hands working with inside.

Chapter 14: Value of Whole Foods And Color Variety

To implement the proper plant-based diet ensure that you consume food items that are as close to being of their original state is possible. A wide range of whole plant food items in the variety of colors you want can be sure you're getting many minerals as well as antioxidants, vitamins amino acids and proteins and phytonutrients. Consuming foods that are colorful, such as fruits and vegetables that are dark in color as well as green tea and fruit can help in reducing the risk of developing disease, speedy recovery, and help protect cell health.

An excellent place to start is eating a variety of fruits and vegetables. I recommend eating one big raw salad per day. It can be loaded with whatever vegetables you would like, then healthy fats such as avocado and hemp seeds can be added. You can also add an element of protein like lentils or edamame, if needed and it can be dressed with Apple cider vinegar and a fat-free dressing.

Make use of the five-ingredient rule

If you see more than five ingredients on the nutrition label this is a clear indication of food that is processed in a way and you should avoid these. This is the most simple and most simple method to prevent impulse buying of the most processed and unhealthy food items.

Stay with whole grain grains.

Whole grain pasta Whole grain pasta, whole grain bread, and whole grain cereals It's easy to see the picture. It is not necessary to get rid of carbs. In fact, you should enjoy them since they are essential to the healthy vegan diet. eating clean is simply about knowing which type of carb is right for you. Whole grains are always a secure option.

Revamp your Food Environment

It's the time to clean out your cabinets. One way to make sure that you don't eat unhealthy food is to remove it from your home entirely. As with all addictions, the best method to eliminate it from the way is to cut it in the early stages.

It isn't possible to eat junk food if there's no food available If it's difficult to drive to the grocery store to grab a snack late at night, you'll ask yourself if it's worthwhile. When you have created an environment that is healthy for food and you become accustomed to the foods that surround you.

It's common for mistakes to happen.

Changes are often difficult and getting rid of unhealthy and addictive food isn't easy for the majority of people. If you do give in and consume junk food on occasion do not blame yourself and quit. In the end, we're humans, it's a cyclical procedure; we are able to make a mistake into an learning experience. Keep in mind that you don't have to be perfect to succeed. Rather, try to make whole food the most important part of your diet slowly , but gradually.

Anti-inflammatory food items

About 12.9 million people across the globe have died due to a cardiovascular condition According to data of the World

Health Organization in 2012. The estimates are that every year, around eight million people die from their lives due to cancer. Heart and cancer will continue to be the leading cause of death in advanced nations that follow a Western diet for years to be.

In order to increase your odds of avoiding these common dangers to your health, it's recommended to include anti-inflammatory foods in your diet. Below are a list of most recommended foods that are vital anti-inflammatory agents.

Fruits, vegetables and starches

As always, we want to choose food items that are colorful. Leafy greens are full of vitamin K and, along with spinach and kale, help reduce inflammation. So do broccoli and cabbage. Additionally, whole grains like brown rice, whole wheat oatmeal, bread and other grains that are not refined are rich in fiber, which can help in reducing inflammation.

Dark leafy greens

Studies have proven that vitamin E plays a significant role in protecting our bodies from inflammation-causing molecules known as Cytokines. One of the best source of the vitamin is dark green vegetables like collard greens, kale and spinach. The dark greens are also known to contain higher levels of vitamins and minerals like calcium, iron, and phytochemicals that fight diseases that counterparts of lighter colors do not have.

Tomatoes

Red tomatoes are high in lycopene, which has been proven to reduce inflammation in the body as well as throughout the lung. Tomatoes cooked well have a higher amount of lycopene than tomatoes that are raw and, therefore, eating tomato sauce can be very beneficial.

Turmeric and ginger

The body uses turmeric by helping to reduce the NF-kappa B, a type of protein that assists in the control of the immune system. It also triggers inflammation. Ginger is, however is proven to reduce intestinal inflammation when taken as supplements.

Berries

They are known as the stars of the medicine and fruit world, berries stand out because of their high levels of antioxidants and fibers, such as quercetin that is an flavonoid which helps to support the growth of healthy intestinal bacteria and helps prevent damage to the colon. The berries have also been found to reduce mental decline and improve memory.

If you're allergic to any items listed It is advised to stay clear of them, regardless of how many nutrients they're packed with. Consuming food that is sensitized to you can create more inflammation rather than reducing it.

A Simple Daily Meal Plan

This means that you're getting an ongoing supply of carbohydrates, proteins, fats and calories you require to perform well. It is not necessary to adhere to the same food plan each day (as repetition could result in being bored very quickly) however, the intention of eating a small portion of six meals and snacks is to remain the same. The aim is to stay away from simple carbs and sugars, while nourish your body and mind with wide range of minerals and vitamins. Mix up your favourite fruits and vegetables grains, nuts, grains, and seeds for a variety of dishes.

The most important thing is to take plenty of water Drink plenty of water! A minimum of one 8oz glass of water with each small meal, and one at the time you get to the world in the early morning and another before you go to bed. Your body requires to stay well-hydrated to function effectively.

Breakfast should consist of of hemp seeds and protein. Make a nutritious smoothie that is made of frozen spinach, bananas, kale and a couple of teaspoons of hemp seeds and any milk that is non-dairy you prefer. If you're craving something more, eat one of your most-loved fruit.

Snack

Consume some nuts for your daily dose of healthy fats. Almonds and walnuts are the ones I'd recommend. If you're looking for something that's more satisfying, try eating nuts and butter (almonds are, as always an excellent option) along with bread made of wheat.

Lunch

Lunch should be a mixture of protein and complex carbohydrates. Take a bite that is brown rice, or quinoa along with sweet potatoes and broccoli. If you've had a snack of nuts instead of butter on bread, you could create a wheat bread sandwich that is filled with hummus, tomatoes, cucumbers, and other vegetables you like. If you're feeling adventurous then you can create your own hummus using chickpeas lemon, tahini and any other spices and serve it as an ingredient for your week's meals.

Dinner

A veggie burger made of black beans served with a salad is a wonderful blend of a nutritious and filling dish. Include a selection of kale, spinach , and lettuce. Add vegetables high in nutrients like tomatoes, beans and carrots. Choose an appropriate dressing that's not heavy in fats, or even butter. You can make your own one using balsamic vinegar as well as a tablespoon of olive oil extra-virgin.

Second snack

Finish the day by eating fresh celery, and the dip of a nut butter that you prefer. Or take a hemp shake. The trick is to eat smaller portions during the course of your day.

To Cut or Bulk?

A lot of people think that protein is needed to build muscles, but this is not the case.

It is suggested to eat the bulk of your protein while you are reducing your weight, as you need to maintain the muscle you've put in when cutting.

For example. If you are eating 1g of protein for every kilogram of bodyweight, as the diet plan we recommend it is necessary to increase that up to 1.5g of protein per kilogram of body weight you weigh in order to reduce your intake.

The calculation of your daily fat intake objective

I recommend that 20%/30 percent of your calories should be comprised of fat. Also, for a more straightforward calculation opt for 20 percent fat.

You are able to make changes according to your needs however I would never exceed 30% or less than 20 percent. For example, my current requirements for daily calories are 2400 calories daily. 20 percent of that's the 480 calories. 9 calories per gram of fat is 53g fat per day.

Calculating your daily carbohydrate needs. The rest of the calories you need to consume should be derived from carbohydrates.

As I typically get 1000 calories from protein, and 480 of my calories from fats so I'd have 920 calories to use to carbs. The 920 calories multiplied by the 4 grams of calories is equal approximately 230 grams carbohydrates every day.

At the end of the day the course, you should be able to calculate your macros with ease.

The most well-known breakdown is protein at 40 percent, fat 20%, carbohydrate 40% - Do not worry that you're off on the exact number as each person is different and you'll find that you need to test and adapt to your needs before you determine what is right for you.

Chapter 15: Bring The Beef on The Chest and Abs

The chest - Weightlifting is most likely the most suggested exercise for people who want to bulk the chest. But, there are those who are looking to build their chest without the barbells that are basic; therefore, here are some exercises to try to achieve a hard-core chest.

Pushups. Now we understand the reason why military plebes were dropping their weight to "giving 50" to satisfy their drill officers achieved that amount of bulk. The secret is in the pushups. This particular exercise is fantastic since you can perform it almost anywhere as long as you have an even surface to perform it on. It is the ideal time for doing a few pushups regardless of whether you are on vacationor at work. (Try this to get rid of your sleepiness. It's effective!) At the home, while watching TV, etc.

Maximize the benefits of your pushups and create your own routine. You can test yourself by doing every pushup you can in the time limit of 30 seconds. Take a deep breath slowly as you lower yourself down to the floor. Exhale as you move back up. Be sure your body is straight and solid during this exercise. Make sure that you do not place your stomach down while you lift your upper body up.

Pushups every two weeks is sure to reveal the muscle of your chest in a short time. Begin by easing into the exercise , and gradually increase the amount. Keep challenging yourself to do more.

Exercises using dumbbells. Two exercises can be done with dumbbells that will aid in strengthening the chest muscle. The first is the flat fly that you lay on the ground with your arms stretched out to either side, in a crucifix like position using dumbbells on both hand. With great control, you lift the dumbbells towards your back while making sure your elbows don't bend as you do so. Two sets of 12 repetitions without rest is suggested to accomplish this.

Another workout that uses dumbbells to strengthen your chest muscle is the bench press. It begins by bringing your return to the bench, feet planted on the floor and the dumbbells straight up to the front of your body. It is a slow process of bringing the dumbbells downwards to your chest and then up again, bringing the two dumbbells of both hands close to one and then the other.

Repeat the exercise until to the point of exhaustion, with no breaks. This exercise is similar to the traditional bench press with the barbell, however this gives more flexibility to the wrists, and is beneficial for people who have had injuries in the past.

The abs are perhaps the most difficult muscle group that need to be toned is your abdominals due to the fact that the midsection is one of the parts of our body that absorbs fat quickly. A week of eating out eventually takes its toll on your stomach, and it is essential to maintain a strict adherence in order willing to tackle the task of shedding those love handles and achieving those infamous "washboard abs."

Two exercises are primarily focused on the midsection. They are crunches and leg raises. any effort to build the most perfect body be incomplete without them. The best part is that you don't have to perform them every day. The trick is to adhere to the proper form and perform these exercises 10 to 30 times , with minimal or no interruption. A good breathing technique can reduce the stress of this exercise.

In case you were not aware that the term "abs" is a shorthand for abdominals.

Crunches: There are many variations to this exercise. But, they all employ the same exercise that involves "crunching" your body forward from a seated position , with the back pointing to the floor. The abdomen is the area that the body bends and the muscles that are located in this region receive the greatest toned from this exercise. The crunches that you do are ideal to build the side and upper muscles of the abdomen.

Leg raises are also great to strengthen the lower muscles of the abdominal region leg raises are your most effective option. This exercise comes with numerous variations, and it can be performed on all fours, or with the back lying flat to the floor. The repetition of stretching the legs strengthens the muscles in the core.

Bicycle crunches. If you're looking to increase the intensity of abdominal exercise it is possible to do the bicycle crunch. It is a combination of both the crunch as well as raising your leg. The process begins by lying down on the floor and then bringing your body so that your right knee is almost touching the left elbow and reverse it in a circular motion. If you can complete 3 to 4 sets with 15-20 repetitions each set every week, then you've achieved your goal.

Chapter 16: The Exercise Routine

As mentioned previously in the previous article, the best exercises are those of the compound type which utilizes the barbell or chin-up bar.

It is important to keep in mind that you require a well-controlled technique. Always ensure that you're working throughout the entire range of motion starting from the lowest to the highest.

Perform these exercises in proper form and technique in your six-repetition range. This is all you have to accomplish. In the end, your body will take on its most natural form. The muscles will all be in the right proportion.

Here's a list of exercise...

Bench press

Incline bench press

Dips

Pressing the barbell on your shoulder standing up

Press your triceps in a standing position

Chin-ups that have a wide grip

Chin-ups reverse close-grips
Barbell curl
Standing squats
Dead lift
Spreading lying scissors
Calf raises
Abdominal crunches
Bicycle is a cruncher

If you think it's not many exercises then you're right. However, you must be aware that many of these exercises exercisers are working multiple muscles simultaneously. All you need is these to build the perfect body for a man.

The exercises are natural in that they train different muscles. For instance, bench press exercises work for the chest area, front deltoids and the triceps. Chin-ups work muscles in the muscles of the lats (the muscles that provide the V-taper) as well as the rear deltoids and the biceps. Squats work the upper legs, the lower back and butt.

You will be working out with each exercise group, at least every week. Thus, you'll be doing three workout sessions per week.

These are the sessions and the exercises you'll be using during every sessions...

Session one

Bench press

Incline bench press

Dips

Barbells for the shoulder press

Press your triceps in a standing position

Session two

Chin-ups with wide grip

Chin-ups reverse close-grips

Barbell curl

Session three

Standing squats

Dead lift

Spreading lying scissors

Calf raises

Buttocks and abdominals must be worked out at the end of every session.

It is important to schedule the time to rest for a day between sessions. Your body requires the time to unwind.

Session one

Bench press

Bench press can be described as the most popular exercise for chest muscles. It mostly targets the middle portion of the.

Be aware that lifting the largest weights are not the ultimate goal. The muscle should be worked to its fullest. The weight should be moved to the bottom position to the highest position.

Do not throw on your chest with the burden. This could result in injuries and also relieve pressure from the muscle.

Throughout the move, keep the arms out in a straight line and align with shoulders.

The movement should be a straight line that runs up and down.

Maintain your shoulders in a neutral position. This will ensure that all your chest muscles engaged.

Place your thumbs on the bar. Do not use a grip that is open to the hand. If you use it, your weight could slide and fall to your chest. This is a frequent occurrence in gyms.

Your feet should be level on your floor. Spread them out wide. This helps keep your body in place. It is not a good idea to fall off the bench while holding the weight of a large piece.

Do not stop at the bottom or at the top, of the exercise. By doing this, you take tension off your muscles. Continue to work without stopping.

The initial position is with the bar placed over the chest, with arms straight up. Lower and then raise it in an upward or down direction. This will help keep the weight level.

Incline bench press

It is designed for strengthen the upper part of the chest.

Do the same in the same way as you would perform the bench press. Only difference lies in in the angle. You should use a bench that allows you to alter the angle of the incline. The angle can be adjusted from 30 and 45 degrees.

Try at moving the body upwards and downwards in the vertical direction. The arms should remain toward the sides throughout the workout.

The position at the bottom should be where the bar is resting against upper quarter of the chest.

Make sure to secure your thumbs on the barbell to avoid slipping.

Dips

This workout strengthens the lower portion of your chest by using parallel bars. Many gyms have them.

Grab the bars and push yourself upwards until your arms are nearly locked. Lower your body to feel a nice stretch through the chest muscle. Without stopping you can push your body up.

Your elbows should naturally flare towards the sides. This will help ensure pressure is applied to the entire chest area below.

This is a difficult exercise. Don't get discouraged even if you only manage only one or two exercises to begin with. You'll soon be able to improve.

The weight of your body will usually suffice to support your weight. If you'd like to add more pounds to the body with belts. You don't want to develop this area too much. Keep it up to six sets per set.

Continue doing sets until you realize that you're not able to do any more than six times.

Barbells for the shoulder press

This is the primary exercise that targets your entire should region. Additionally, it strengthens the triceps.

Clean the weight off the floor, or off the rack for squatting.

Take the bar in the bar in a closed grip with the thumbs wrapped around bar. This helps to prevent any slippage from the bar.

The ideal starting point is to have the weight on the upper chest. From there, push the weight up straight upwards.

In the final part of the move, you should push your hips to the side and then pull your chest back. This allows the weight to move past your forehead and chin. If the weight begins to rise above your head, lift your hips back to a position. Repeat this hip and chest motion while you lower the weight.

Make sure you shift the weight throughout the entire motion, starting from starting from the lowest point to the straightest position of your arms.

Do not stop either at the bottom or the top. Maintain your speed.

Pressing the triceps while standing

This exercise targets on the entire triceps region.

Be sure to use the full range of movement. It should be easy to feel the complete stretch near the end of the motion.

Begin by putting the weight on top of your head. Again, hold the bar using a tight grip to prevent the bar from sliding.

Lower the weight back behind your head, bending your arms. Make sure to keep your upper body straight and pointed upwards throughout the entire workout.

Keep your eyes straight while you are performing your exercises. If you look upwards you could cause injury to the neck's back.

This concludes session one. In this workout you've worked your shoulders, chest and the triceps muscles.

Session two

There are only two exercises for your back in this workout. These exercises target all over the back.

The lower back should already have been strengthened by exercises such as dead-lifts and squats. These exercises will be covered in the third session.

Chin-ups with wide grip

Find the Chin-up bar. These are available in virtually every fitness center.

This workout targets the lats. They're the muscles which create that tapered look.

If you begin this exercise it is likely that you will discover it difficult. Try every repetition you're able. You'll improve.

If you are unable to do one rep, try placing your legs on cushion to aid you. Make use of a sturdy chair or box. When you are stronger, you'll be able to quit using this.

If you want you wanted to, you can add mass to your physique. But, you'll discover that your body weight is sufficient.

Reduce your repetitions to 6 per set. Repeat sets until you realize that you aren't with perfect form.

To hold the bar in the proper length, lift your arms high and bend at a straight angle. The ideal position is to have your arms at a level with your shoulders in the middle and your forearms pointed toward the sky. The hands' width is now at the ideal length for this workout. Hold the bar in the same width. This will allow you to stretch the lats completely.

Begin each repetition with a pull your shoulders downwards. This will activate your back muscles completely. It will ensure that your back muscles are performing the job. If not, your arms could take on too much of the task.

As with any exercise, perform the entire range of motion. When you reach the bottom of the exercise your shoulders should be stretched to the max. When you reach high point of move attempt to reach the bar to at the very top of your chest. It's irrelevant if fail to make it. By trying to reach the chest, you'll ensure that you're the highest you can.

If you exercise the entire range of motion it will be sure that you're working your entire muscle group.

Chin-ups reverse close grips

This exercise makes use of your biceps and triceps, and is more effective in hitting the middle of your back region.

Begin with gripping your bar with the shoulder length. Use an underhand grip. This means that you should have your palms facing forward while you grip the bar.

In the wide-grip chin-up begin the exercise by pulling the back and then down using your shoulders. This will ensure that your back is properly engaged.

Always aim for all of your range of motion. Extend your muscles to the bottom, and then pull upwards as high as you can.

Barbell curl

This exercise will help strengthen the biceps across their entire length.

Begin by placing the barbell placed on the floor directly in your face.

Take the bar in the bar's shoulder width, under-handed grip at. Place your thumbs on the bar to keep it from sliding.

Get up to ensure that the bar hangs on your upper thighs.

The bar should be moved to your shoulders, following an arcuate arc. Keep your upper arms steady and to the side during the entire movement. Don't swing the bar upwards using your arms or by swinging your body. Only move the lower arms.

Utilize the entire flexibility of your body using straight arms to the bottom and arms bent fully to the upper.

In this workout the back muscles are worked muscles, shoulders, and biceps.

Session three

This workout focuses on lower back and the legs.

Standing squats

This workout targets the upper legs. It also targets muscles in the buttocks (butt) as well as the low back muscles.

Make use of the Squat rack. Do not use an equipment. The machine limits movement and prevents the body to move along its natural course. This means that your muscles don't grow fully.

Begin by placing the barbell upon the rack for squatting. If you begin by placing your weight lying on the ground, you might be having trouble getting it back towards your shoulders.

The ideal height is one that is aligned with the top of your chest. This will help you keep your feet level on the ground when you lift the bar off.

While facing the bar, step beneath so that the bar is placed on the shoulder's top. Make sure that it is below your neck. The weight placed on your neck is likely to cause injuries.

Your feet should be shoulder-width apart, with the feet slightly pointing towards the outside.

Grab the bar with your the shoulder length. This will help to keep your shoulders tight and ensure that the bar will be supported on your back. Utilize an overhand grip with thumbs placed on the top. Maintain the weight tightly against the upper shoulder region.

Once you are it is time to move two feet back. This should be 4 to 6 feet from where the rack is.

Straighten your back and then push your chest forward. Avoid looking up. This can result in neck injuries. Be sure to keep looking straight ahead through the exercise. This will help ensure alignment and help prevent injuries.

The barbell should be moved in a straight, straight up and down direction throughout the exercise. Try to hold the barbell above toes in the middle while you go up and down. Be sure to ensure that your knees don't go more forward than your feet. Maintain your back straight with your keep your chest lifted.

In the lower part, you should aim for that your hips are a little less than your knees. Keep knees slightly pointing towards the side, just over your feet. Maintain your back straight when leaning forward to about 45 degrees. This will ensure that the weight stays over the middle of your foot. From here, you'll continue to move up, while keeping the barbell in the same position directly over in the center of your foot.

It's recommended to practice the exercise with no weights. In this way, you can be sure that you're doing it right.

Dead lift

Begin with the bar placed on the floor. Your feet should be just a little narrower than the shoulder width, with your toes pointed out. Place the bar in mid-foot. Make sure to keep this position for the entire exercise.

Grab your bar using both hands with your palms facing forwards. Your thumbs should be curled over the bar in order to prevent sliding. Use a shoulder-width grasp on the bar.

You can lift the bar up by straightening it upwards. Keep your back straight with your chest up, and look forward throughout the entire movement. Do not arch your back, since this can cause injuries. Utilize the entire range of motion from the floor down to the floor, and all the way back up.

Calve raises

This is a workout for all muscles of the calf. Lift a barbell to arms ' length. Set yourself on a platform which is about three inches tall. Place the soles of your feet placed on the block, and your remaining feet elevated above the floor.

Keep your body straight move the body using your legs up and down. Do a stretch to the bottom of the exercise.

Do sets of six repetitions.

In this exercise you've worked your lower back and leg muscles.

Chapter 17: Finding and Maintaining

The Right Attitude

People around the world aren't the same! There are various cultures, races characteristics, attitudes, and behaviours. However, we all want to believe that we are distinctive "in reality, we are distinctive!"

How can we develop an the universally good character and attitude that can help us get through the tough times and be the most effective of us?

This chapter we'll look at some methods that are effective to address the earlier question.

As I stated above, we are unique! Sure , we may share the same values as our neighbors. But in the personal, we are certainly different.

Every person is unique with their genes, as well as their perspective of themselves and their environment.

This can lead to different strategies for managing our anger, desires, dreams and the rest of life.

What's the best way the mindset that will aid us in keeping up with the fitness world and remain physically active? !

Self-image and self-esteem:

You may have heard, self-image is how you view yourself. It could be the way you view your body, what kind of persona you possess, or what people think of you, just to name a some. Self-esteem refers to how you consider yourself.

Self-image and self-esteem are closely related! If you're not happy with your self-image, then you'll not feel comfortable in your body and that can result in you have a low self-esteem.

If you have issues with your self-image and self-esteem can hinder your efforts to stay physically active and achieving your goals.

Now you may be asking yourself: How can I increase my self-image and self-esteem? !

The first thing to do is acknowledge that there isn't an instant solution that can instantly improve self-image and self-esteem! It is a determination to work on it regularly.

Being honest with ourselves may be the first step in the right direction. You know your own, most of your flaws and most of your strengths.

The best methods to boost self-image and self-esteem are:

Understanding ourselves;

Accept constructive criticism from the people around us;

Accept our positive qualities;

Find ways to strengthen our abilities;

Make a list of things you admire about yourself, including the way you present yourself, your personality, and your skills

Find internet research on the topic of self-image and self-esteem

Find books on the subject.

Participate in seminars as often as you can.

Confidence:

Confidence is influenced by our accomplishments and the sense that we are part of something, and our self-esteem. In addition, our accomplishments as well as our sense of identity can have an effect on our self-esteem.

In other words , confidence is a realistic view of the self and abilities of one's own.

It's good to know that that confidence is learned, not passed down through the generations!

The level of confidence not the same for each one! On the other hand, there are those who have a great level of confidence. They believe in their capabilities to achieve things by making plans and being prepared to overcome obstacles. In addition, even the fact that they do not achieve certain objectives, they remain optimistic and find ways to reenergize their motivation and gain knowledge from their mistakes.

In the opposite,, we have those who are unsure. The lack of confidence may result from a number of factors from childhood, repeated previous failures, the impact of society, the culture, and a myriad of other reasons. But, the lack confidence needs to be taken care of.

In the end, just like self-image and self-esteem, increasing confidence takes time commitment, dedication and persistence.

These are the characteristics of people who are confident:

Self-love

Self belief;

They can be comfortable in themselves.

Self-awareness;

Fearlessness;

Experiment;

Happiness

Achieving a High-Performance State of Mind:

In the previous paragraph, I briefly discussed some details about self-image confidence and self-esteem. Since these elements play an important part in the ability of a person to achieve the desired results and also to remain physically active.

How can we get the mindset that allows us to exercise without having to relapse after a few months or even weeks? or how can we attain the state of mind that reenergizes us and help us get out of the plateau?

Before beginning bodybuilding one must first deal with the issues within themselves that could prevent them from achieving their goals. The best method to truly find motivation to keep it going and rekindle it is to think about What are the motivations that have me deciding to begin this new chapter in my life?

The answers to the question can range from the physical benefits to being active to personal reasons! !

Personally, I'd suggest taking the time to take a break in a location you love. It is important to be thinking about the place! If you're thinking that you want to have a particular design "A authentic one" Close your eyes and imagine how great you'll feel in your skin after being you're in the shape. Close your eyes and imagine other goals. The aim of this exercise is to build powerful emotions that can help you along your journey.

However, you may be in an issue of plateau. It is recommended to reduce the amount of workout, and set yourself on a simple "cycle" like three weeks of a simple workout in the midst of a weeks of exercise tubing". I assume that, as an intermediate bodybuilder, you already know the idea of periodicization.

The biggest mistake people make when confronted with the problem of a plateau is that they try to increase the duration and intensity of their time in the fitness center! It will only result in general fatigue and injury.

In the end, by achieving an improvement over time in our self-image, self-esteemand self-esteem, making a list of short - and long-term objectives and establishing an expectation of satisfaction, can help us along our journey. A side note, your system of satisfaction could involve rewarding yourself when you make progress or achieve your goal or simply having an amazing exercise routine. It could be a thing you do each month or every week but it is a personal choice. Furthermore, by making fitness a habit, it will be a part of your daily routine.

Conclusion

Next, you must research further, to better inform yourself to be aware of exactly what you're doing while you move through this course.

Begin by understanding your strengths, weaknesses and weaknesses. Work out in order to bring any difficulties to a minimum. Do a test by lifting handful of weights and observing the moment you feel pain. Explore different machines. Which are you most comfortable with, and or do you find yourself avoiding? Are certain treadmills more challenging than others? Do treadmills challenge your balance? Do the results come out good or negative? If left unaddressed, can the sensation of being extremely awkward result in a loss of balance that could result in falling? Consider this as a warning and look for a machine that feels more comfortable or develop an exercise program that aims to improve your balance.

If it's uncomfortable, then you aren't going to perform it. You should make it as easy as possible for yourself and you'll be more likely to do the workout. Once you're comfortable with the routines and equipment make an exercise plan that includes the advice you read inside this publication. Consult your physician to make sure that you're ready for this type of training. Also, ensure you are aware of the medications you're taking. Also examine your diet. Be sure to include sufficient protein. Be sure to follow it with care.